Praise for *The Compassionate Mind Approach to Overcoming Anxiety*

'Learning to treat yourself with kindness and compassion is like learning to ice your feet firmly on the ground. If you are going to walk out of your struggle with anxiety, you need to regain your psychological footing, and this book will show you how. In a gentle, wise and step-by-step way, it will help you establish self-compassion as a habit of mind, and bring that healing quality to your thoughts and actions. Highly recommended.'

Steven C. Hayes, author of *Get Out of Your Mind and Into Your Life*

'...ch writes with warmth and wisdom – as if he is speaking directly to you. He shows how compassion, mindfulness and facing the difficulties of anxiety can bring personal growth. Filled with specific and powerful techniques, readers will find a new path to follow with a brilliant and compassionate guide. I highly recommend this book for all who suffer from anxiety.'

Robert L. Leahy, Ph.D., author of *The Worry Cure*; Director, The American Institute for Cognitive Therapy; Clinical Professor of Psychology, Weill-Cornell University Medical College

'...y to read, grounded in solid research and filled with useful exercises, ...ook is a godsend for those who suffer from anxiety.'

...in Neff, PhD, author of *Self-Compassion*; Associate Professor, University of Texas at Austin

'A superb introduction to a revolutionary new way of dealing with anxiety. The reader is led on a compelling exploration of how the anxious mind works, followed by masterful exercises that tap our innate capacity for comfort and healing – self-compassion. Seamlessly integrating important research and extensive clinical experience, the author speaks through the

pages with the wise, gentle voice of experience. Go ahead – try it and see what happens!'

Christopher K. Germer, PhD, Clinical Instructor, Harvard Medical School; author of *The Mindful Path to Self-Compassion*; Faculty, Institute for Meditation and Psychotherapy

'Cognitive Behaviour Therapy (CBT) has led the way in creating solid science-based treatments. Traditionally, CBT has been an action-oriented treatment. And that action orientation has produced a lot of benefits. More recently, CBT has begun to include more acceptance, mindfulness and self-compassion focused work. Dennis Tirch is a master of both where CBT has been and of where CBT is going. In this book, you will find a broad contemporary understanding of anxiety and a host of very, very practical ways to come into a more compassionate and effective relationship with anxiety. The book offers a different way of being with anxiety that will have implications in your life that extend well beyond anxiety. You can expect changes in your relationship with anxiety that offer a path to rich and engaged living.'

Kelly G. Wilson PhD, co-founder of Acceptance and Commitment Therapy; author of *Things Might Go Terribly, Horribly Wrong*; Associate Professor, University of Mississippi

'Writing in an informative, highly engaging manner, Dr Tirch shares his considerable wisdom in both compassion-based practices and behaviour therapy. The reader is given practical and powerful tools for cultivating a sense of self-compassion in the face of anxiety. A genuine pleasure to read.'

Douglas Mennin, Associate Professor, CUNY Hunter College

THE COMPASSIONATE MIND APPROACH TO OVERCOMING ANXIETY

DENNIS TIRCH

ROBINSON

Constable & Robinson Ltd
55–56 Russell Square
London WC1B 4HP
www.constablerobinson.com

First published in the UK by Robinson,
an imprint of Constable & Robinson Ltd, 2012

A copy of the British Library Cataloguing in
Publication data is available from the British Library

Important Note

This book is not intended as a substitute for medical advice or treatment.
Any person with a condition requiring medical attention should consult
a qualified medical practitioner or suitable therapist.

ISBN 978-1-84901-513-4

Printed and bound in the UK

1 3 5 7 9 10 8 6 4 2

Contents

Part II:
Compassionate Mind Training for Anxiety

Preface

When we experience fear or disappointment, dread or loss we naturally tend to look for support and guidance from those we care about, and who care about us. We turn to them for their acceptance, their understanding and their love. Indeed, the evolution of human behaviour demonstrates how this tendency has emerged in the lifecycle and how we have become able to keenly detect threats in our environment while at the same time abiding in a state of calm through our experience of the support and loving kindness of those around us. Research has shown that from the day that we are born and throughout our lives the kindness of others will have a huge impact on how our brains mature, how our bodies work and on our emotions and general well-being.[1] It has also been shown that treating ourselves with compassion has a huge impact on the quality of our lives and how we deal with difficulties such as anxiety.[2]

It makes sense that we are calmed by the warmth, compassion and connection with others, and that we can also develop healthier ways of responding to life's struggles by directing compassion and kindness inwards, to the way we feel about ourselves.

Our lives can feel so overwhelming, and can be so very short. In the presence of a variety of fearful challenges along our journeys, such as sickness, aging, and the finitude of life, can we direct accepting, open, and warm feelings towards ourselves? If we are capable of such acts, what is the effect? By standing as a compassionate witness to our own pain, can we better be present to our experience, and develop healthier, more fluid ways of responding to life's struggles? This 'self-compassion' may be the foundation for a more flexible, healthy and rewarding life.[3] This book aims to help you do this, and help you understand the nature of your anxiety, the best ways of dealing with it, and how your mind can help you cope with it.

Introduction
by Professor Paul Gilbert

We have always understood that compassion is very important for our well-being. If you are feeling stressed or upset it is always better to have kind, helpful and supportive people around you rather than critical, rejecting or disinterested folk. It is not only commonsense, however, that tells us about the value of kindness and compassion – recent advances in the scientific study of compassion and kindness have greatly advanced our understanding of how compassionate qualities of the mind really do influence our brains, bodies and social relationships, as well as affecting our health and well-being. Yet despite this commonsense ancient wisdom and new knowledge, we live in an age that can make compassion difficult for ourselves and others. This is a world of striving for the competitive edge, of achievement and desire, of comparison to others who are perhaps doing better, leading to dissatisfaction and self-criticism. Research has now revealed that such environments actually make us unhappier, and that mental ill-health is on the increase, especially in younger people. As Dr Dennis Tirch helps us understand, anxiety is a very common symptom of the environments we are living in today.

As if feeling anxious and stressed is not enough, we can also become fearful of these emotions and try to suppress or avoid them, even becoming self-critical for feeling 'overly anxious'. Indeed, our society has a habit of blaming and shaming if we seem to be struggling with our emotions. People with the *right stuff* are not supposed to be anxious, or feel overwhelmed. So anxiety must be an indication that the something wrong with us. Rather than seeing it as an understandable, if undesirable, response to the world in which we live, we blame ourselves for feeling anxious.

So, why are we so susceptible to anxiety and why might anxiety be on the increase in modern society? Dr Tirch uses his wealth of experience and knowledge to guide our understanding and help us recognize that actually many of our emotions are the result of a very long evolutionary history. Our emotions were originally developed to help us deal with rapid threats in the jungles and savannas and are not so well adapted for the modern world. Nor do they do so well when we bring our advanced brains and greater capacity for thinking and rumination to bear on our anxiety. Humans are the only animals that have the ability to worry about tomorrow, or if they have cancer, or are about to have a heart attack, or if others like them. So the way we think about the stresses in our lives can at times really 'do our heads in'. And, of course, we can also think about our internal worlds – the fantasies, thoughts and feelings we have within us. Again, no other animal can do this. Realizing this and being able to stand back from it all allows us to understand that our vulnerability to anxiety is not our fault. After all, we didn't design our brains with their various capacities for emotions such as anxiety and anger. Nor did we design our brain's capacity for complex thinking, which can actually make our experience of anxiety more intense. And we didn't choose our backgrounds or our genes, both of which can make us more susceptible to anxiety. This is a very important message in Compassionate Mind Training and Compassion Focused Therapy, because compassion begins with a deep understanding of just how tricky our brains are and a recognition that they are not that well put together! Once we recognize how difficult our emotions can be, we can stand back from them and feel compassion for the difficulties we experience.

So, given that our brains have evolved and been shaped by the environments we live in, what can we do to help ourselves when we become anxious? First, we can learn to pay attention to how our minds work and function, and become mindful and observant of the feelings that are associated with anxiety. In this very helpful book, Dr Tirch shows how people have learned to be sensitive to feelings of anxiety and, at times, have also learned to be frightened of those feelings.

If we are to face anxiety and work with it then our relationship with ourselves is very important. If we are critical and harsh with ourselves, then our inner worlds are not comfortable places to inhabit. Feeling ashamed

and being self-critical, self-condemning or even self-loathing can undermine our confidence and make us feel bad. Sadly, when things go wrong
and we make mistakes, many of us are self-critical rather than helpful
and supportive of ourselves, and when we feel distressed we react by
becoming frustrated and angry. This is not, in fact, a good way to deal
with anxiety because, as Dr Tirch outlines, you are actually adding more
fuel to the fire of your threat system. In contrast, self-compassion is a
way of being with ourselves in all our emotions, uncomfortable as they
may be, without self-condemning and instead with support and encouragement. Research shows that the more compassionate we are towards
ourselves, the happier we are and the more resilient we become when
faced with difficult events in our lives. In addition, we are better able to
reach out to others for help, and feel more compassionate towards other
people, too.

Compassion can sometimes be viewed as being a bit 'soft' or 'weak' or
'letting your guard down' and 'not trying hard enough'. This is a major
mistake because, on the contrary, compassion requires us to be open to
and tolerant of our painful feelings, and to face up to our own problematic emotions and difficulties. Compassion does not mean turning away
from emotional difficulties or discomforts, or trying to get rid of them.
It is *not* a soft option. Rather, compassion provides us with the courage,
honesty and commitment to learn to cope with the difficulties we face
and alleviates our anxiety. It enables us to do things that help us to flourish and take care of ourselves – not as a demand or requirement, but to
enable us to live our lives more fully and contentedly.

In this book, Dr Tirch offers his many years of experience as a clinical
psychologist, psychotherapist and long-time meditator working in New
York with people experiencing a variety of different emotional difficulties. He also brings his experience of using Compassion Focused Therapy
in the treatment of anxiety. He outlines a model of compassion that seeks
to stimulate and build your confidence so that you can engage with your
anxiety. You will learn how to develop a real, supportive friendship
with yourself that will help you through difficult times. Dr Tirch guides
you to develop compassionate motivations, compassionate attention,

compassionate feelings, compassionate thinking and compassionate behaviour. You will learn about the potential power of developing compassionate imagery that focuses on creating a compassionate sense of yourself and that draws on your own inner wisdom and benevolent qualities – qualities you are most likely to feel when you're feeling calm and/or showing concern for others. Learning how to breathe, to 'slow down' and also to engage with these qualities can be very helpful when anxiety crashes through us like a storm. Using different compassionate images, you will discover that your compassion focus can be visual or aural (e.g. imagining a compassionate voice speaking to you when you need it), and can be especially useful in enabling us to get in touch with our internal compassionate feelings and desires at times of distress.

The approach that Dr Tirch takes is called a Compassionate *Mind* Approach because when we engage compassion it can influence our attention, thoughts, feelings and behaviour – in other words, how our mind operates *as a whole*. The Compassionate Mind Approach outlined in this book draws on many other well-developed approaches, including those of Eastern traditions such as Buddhism. In addition, Compassionate Mind Approaches, especially those that form part of Compassion Focused Therapy, are rooted in scientific understanding of how our mind works. Undoubtedly over the years our understanding of the brain will change and advance. One thing that doesn't change, however, is the fact that kindness, warmth and understanding go a long way towards helping us. In these pages you will find these qualities in abundance so you, too, can learn to be gentle, understanding, supportive and kind but also engaging and courageous when working with your anxiety.

Many people suffer silently and secretly with a whole range of anxiety problems – some feeling ashamed or angry with themselves, others sometimes fearful of anxiety getting the upper hand. Sadly, shame stops many of us from reaching out for help. But, by opening your heart to compassion, you can take the first steps towards dealing with your anxieties in new ways. My compassionate wishes go with you on your journey.

Professor Paul Gilbert, PhD FBPsS OBE

August 2011

A Personal Story and Acknowledgements

Before we go further, let me share with you how this book came into being. As it happens, my personal connection to training in mindfulness, acceptance and compassion began long before I became a psychologist. As a child, at about the age of ten, I was lucky enough to learn the basics of Buddhist meditation from an uncle who had served as a paratrooper in the Second World War. He discovered that Zen Buddhism helped him cope with the harrowing experiences he had witnessed. I suppose he must have noticed how anxious and curious I was, and he began to teach me *zazen*, a form of Japanese meditation that relates to the practice of mindfulness, which is a way of staying in the present moment as deliberately and as fully as possible and which partly involves paying attention to your breathing, moment by moment. I noticed that even when my uncle recalled the sadness and insanity of his wartime experience, his face was graced with a slight smile, and that he seemed to be full of love and kindness. It impressed me so much that I set upon the path that leads to the book you are holding.

In my early twenties, after completing a degree in philosophy and humanities, my attention again turned to an understanding of how Buddhist thought and mind-training exercises could help alleviate suffering. These were the days before 'mindfulness' and 'acceptance' had become trendy terms in Western psychotherapy. My own meditative practice and studies led me to wonder how mindfulness and compassion could be skilfully applied in a modern, Western context. I had no idea how to accomplish this.

After a fair amount of soul searching, I enrolled in graduate school to study psychology. Eventually, I began a PhD course in clinical psychology, with a vision of integrating what I had learned from Buddhist mental training with state-of-the-art Western scientific psychology. I soon realized that the most exciting and effective research and clinical work in psychotherapy was happening at the cutting edge of cognitive behavioural therapy (CBT), which was emerging as a major, effective therapy for a range of difficulties including anxiety. I spent a great deal of time cross-referencing CBT principles with those found in Mahayana Buddhism, and envisioning an effective, practical therapy that would use both methods.

On the horizon, and about to enter the field of CBT, other psychologists were starting to explore adaptations of Buddhist contemplative thought as alternative forms of behaviour therapy. Throughout the 1990s a psychologist named Steven Hayes and a number of his colleagues were developing Acceptance and Commitment Therapy (ACT),[1] which involved learning to accept thoughts and emotions as they arise and living in accordance with our deepest values. Marsha Linehan, a psychologist and student of Zen Buddhism, developed Dialectical Behaviour Therapy (DBT)[2] for people with turbulent emotions who might be prone to suicide attempts. Both ACT and DBT merged Eastern and Western psychologies, and amassed a strong body of research that provided a sound base of evidence for their effectiveness.

When I was at graduate school, something else happened that profoundly affected me: my father died from diabetes. The disease caused his death to be slow and the process was regrettably difficult for him; however, during his illness I was able to visit him while he was in hospital. He was always dignified during this time, and talked to me of many things, including his guilt over things he had done, or not done, and of his pain. He was also hoping for some kind of redemption or absolution before his life ended, and he was filled with anxiety. He needed compassion, and I felt it was one of the most important things, indeed perhaps the only thing, I would be able to give him. This experience, however dreadful and sad, allowed me to understand the way compassion could bring peace, restfulness and calm to a worried, anxious mind.

During my internship and post-doctoral training two factors brought me into much closer contact with the power of acceptance, compassion and applied mindfulness, which can be understood as the non-judgemental observation of the contents of consciousness mindfulness that works hand in hand with compassion to help us develop a non-judgemental awareness of ourselves. As we work with our habitual tendency to judge our thoughts and feelings, we are working towards the development of mindfulness, which in turn helps us to cultivate self-compassion. Mindfulness and compassion are related but separate processes. But the of the two factors that brought me close to the practice of mindfulness, the first was personal: our training director, Dr Richard Amodio, and I spent many hours walking through the green, rural campus of the Bedford Massachusetts Veterans Affairs Medical Center, where we discussed a variety of ways that mindfulness and compassion could be used in psychotherapy. As a result, we designed and piloted a group treatment for Vietnam-era veterans of heavy combat trauma. This pilot programme brought us into contact with clients who taught us a great deal about the power of compassion and self-forgiveness, and I believe we were all changed through the process of treatment.

The second factor to influence me was the absolute explosion in research and publishing involving CBT and mindfulness. The field of study we were involved with seemed to change and expand each week. As a result, I immersed myself in the academic literature; what I learned transformed my life's work and ultimately led me to the practise of Compassion Focused Therapy (CFT), on which this book is based.

For the past nine years I have worked with Dr Robert Leahy at The American Institute for Cognitive Therapy, where I serve as Associate Director. Our institute is an internationally known CBT practice, and a centre of training for psychology graduate students, professionals and post-doctoral residents. Dr Leahy is a well-known master clinician and a prolific writer in the field of CBT; he has a broad perspective that takes in a range of psychological insights and discoveries. Over several years, Dr Leahy and I have been engaged in an active research programme to examine the relationships between people's beliefs about their emotions and their capacity for mindfulness and acceptance, as well as for many other variables.[3]

I've been fortunate to attend a number of residential and intensive trainings led by a range of teachers such as Steven Hayes, Kelly Wilson,

Zindel Segal, Chris Germer and Robyn Walser. I've also been grateful to be involved in the development of a growing ACT community in New York City. We have been steadily developing new opportunities for therapists who are seeking training in mindfulness and acceptance-based therapy. During this time, my consultation with Kelly Wilson has been particularly important to developing an understanding of how fundamental behavioural processes can unfold into the awe-inspiring human capacity for compassion.

Along with this scientific study, some of my most profound lessons have taken place in spiritual contexts, such as my ongoing work with Buddhist and Central Asian meditation traditions, and on extended music and meditation retreats led by the English guitarist, Robert Fripp. Currently, my personal spiritual studies have returned to Zen yoga and Tibetan Buddhism; however, I have found that all forms of meditative and psychotherapy practice I have encountered have had their usefulness. There are certain principles regarding how we can interact with our inner selves and the world around us in ways that contribute to our well-being. At the heart of these principles, again and again, is the importance of compassion.

In the middle of this activity, some six years ago, Dr Leahy introduced me to Professor Paul Gilbert, a good friend of his. This introduction radically affected my professional and personal life; Professor Gilbert is a master of the topics of evolutionary psychology and neuroscience of emotion and is also deeply involved in exploring how Buddhist concepts such as compassion and mindfulness can be used outside the bounds of strictly spiritual settings and linked to modern psychological science. He has done a great deal of work on shame and self-criticism, and has found that people who are prone to feeling shameful and critical of themselves also have a hard time being open to the compassion of others and to the idea of developing self-compassion,[4] which they see as a weakness or even something to be frightened of. So, compassion, and especially developing self-compassion, became a key focus for his work, because evidence was pointing to the fact that our brains work much more efficiently and are much more able to remain on an even keel if we surround ourselves with others who are kind, supportive and compassionate.[5]

When I began to read Paul's work, I had the sense that many threads of my professional life were being woven together in his new approach: Compassion Focused Therapy (CFT), which builds on the insights and developments of a variety of fields in psychotherapy but in particular on CBT. It draws on what research is telling us about how our brains process emotion, the way our brains have evolved to require certain social inputs, and it draws on Eastern psychology's history of mind training. Paul believes, as I do, that before you can fix something you need to know how it works, and that can only come from the science. We began to correspond and collaborate and for a number of subsequent years CFT became a central aspect of my own clinical work, research and writing.

After working on a chapter and an article together, I visited Paul in Derby in the UK to take part in his training, and to discuss CFT in greater depth. I was accompanied by Dr Russell Kolts, who is now studying and writing about how compassionate mind training can help patients overcome problems with anger and uncontrollable rage. I was fascinated by the possibilities that CFT provided, and the time spent with Paul and Russell again broadened my perspective to the humbling, healing power of mindful compassion. It was when I was with them the idea for the book emerged. I have been very lucky to build a relationship with Paul and with Russell, who have fuelled my dedication to this work.

I would like to acknowledge the groundbreaking work on self-compassion that has been conducted by Kristin Neff and Christopher Germer, as well as the significant advances in CFT applications that have been made by Lynne Henderson and Kenn Goss. They are part of a growing community within psychological science that understands the importance of compassion in our well-being. Of course, I am deeply grateful for the help of the editors of this book, Professor Paul Gilbert and Fritha Saunders. I would also like to take a moment to recognize the wisdom and compassion that I have learnt from clients, closest colleagues, students and my family; John,

Leah, Lily, Neal and Jaclyn, as well as my mother Janet, truly my first teacher in compassion.

How This Book is Structured

If you are holding this book it is likely you have had some trouble with anxiety at some point in your life. My hope is that the practices I will describe will open the way to greater self-compassion, well-being, and a growing capacity to bring mindful awareness and kindness into your life, moment by moment.

It may be useful for you to have a pen and paper or special notebook nearby so that you can record any observations you may have as you read this book and so that you can complete or copy some of the practical exercises that have been included.

This book is divided into two sections: Part I provides background information that explores the evolutionary nature of anxiety and how it operates. Part II examines how we are able to soothe our anxiety by experiencing a sense of safety, contentment and calm. We will learn of the sometimes-untapped capacities we have to alleviate our anxiety using our intuitive wisdom, courage and compassion. Part II also provides detailed, workable and user-friendly techniques based on CFT to help you overcome your anxiety. The most significant techniques in this section are called 'Compassionate Mind Training', which aim to help you balance the way you regulate your emotions and in particular (but not exclusively) stimulate the system in your brain that helps you feel safe and connected (what we call 'affiliated') with others and with your own compassionate self.

CFT uses imagery and visualization techniques adapted from Buddhist practices as well from modern CBT techniques. It is deeply important if, during this process, you imagine having a very good friend with you – one who cares completely about you and wants to see you prosper.

In CFT we talk a lot about building our capacity for compassion. What this means is that we prepare ourselves for the work we are going to do; for example, if you want to run a marathon then you will train for it gradually and deliberately, rather than decide to do it one day and then run it the next. Developing our ability to accept, regulate and cope with our anxiety follows a similar course of training.

The aim of Part II is to provide a practical, reliable and repeatable programme to help you develop a compassionate mind when you feel anxious or distressed.

Dennis Tirch, 2011

Part I

The Compassionate Mind Approach to Overcoming Anxiety

1 The Emergence of Anxiety

Anxiety is one of the most common problems that people face. The potential is everywhere, be it applying for a new job, taking exams, or meeting new people. You won't be surprised when I tell you that working as a cognitive behavioural psychotherapist in the heart of mid-town Manhattan, I've spent a lot of time in the presence of a wide variety of different types of anxiety. Manhattan is a busy metropolitan city that can seem rather obsessed with getting things done and it is crowded with people hurrying along the streets. It is easy to imagine the almost mythical promise of opportunity, laced with the experience of lightning-paced stress, linked to expectations and deadlines. Just outside my window, the pavements are heaving with ambitious men and women in business suits and fashionable hipsters chatting or texting into mobiles, all rushing about their lives in pursuit of their goals. Even if you close your eyes, the pulsing sound of the traffic, the occasional siren, the beeping horns and the constant hum of activity reverberates through the windows and walls.

It was in this city, packed into a crowded subway car, that one of my clients, who we'll call Jennifer, first encountered the depth and intensity of her own experience of anxiety. Jennifer was deeply committed to her work as a pre-school teacher and her heartfelt dedication to help young children had been what she'd wanted to do for as long as she could remember. As she sat on the subway one morning, with every one of her lessons carefully planned and her smartphone with her schedule in perfect order, her life seemed to be in control. Jennifer had high standards for herself, and was a caring and conscientious person. I would imagine that her students and their families were lucky to have such a teacher in their lives.

But that particular morning, as she looked around at the densely packed fellow passengers who were surrounding her, and felt the clacking, vibrating movement of the train, Jennifer began to feel as if it were difficult to take a deep breath. This seemed odd, and worrisome. She began to pay close attention to this strange sensation, and as she did, her chest began to feel tight and constricted.

'Oh, God,' she thought, 'what is happening? Am I freaking out or something? Am I coming down with the flu?'

Suddenly, she felt trapped, as if the train were closing in on her, with no possibility of escape. As these thoughts began to race through her mind, she continued to frantically check for signs that she was becoming ill, or worse. She grew dizzy, and began to panic. Her brow began to bead with sweat, and she told herself, 'I need to get out of here! What if I can't escape? Get me out.' Startling herself, she began to cry. She covered her face, and as soon as the train reached the next stop she pushed her way through the thick cluster of other exiting passengers and ran up the stairs to the level of the street.

As she emerged into daylight and fresh air, Jennifer was still far from her stop, and this meant that she would certainly be late for work. Disorientated, she looked around for a taxi, but there were none to be found. Waves of shame and embarrassment moved through her: she didn't understand how she could have 'lost control' so intensely, so suddenly. Worries about being fired, or chided in front of her colleagues for her lateness percolated in her imagination. Stunned, she barely managed to straighten her typically perfectly pressed and professional clothes and make her way to school. Although she felt mortified to make the call, later that day she contacted my office and sought help for what she felt was potentially crippling anxiety. I can clearly recall our first telephone chat; every word she spoke seemed steeped in fear and self-criticism. Jennifer did not seem to be kind and understanding of her painful experience; instead she asked herself: 'How could this have happened to me when I am so very careful, and have worked so hard to be in control? What's wrong with me? Am I going crazy? Have I lost it? Could anything help?' This was not the first time she had felt trapped and panicked, and the fear of there being something wrong with her, and that it was out of her control seemed to spin her around in spirals of anxiety.

Over the course of a year, Jennifer and I worked together to help her deal with what proved to be severe panic attacks and chronic worries. In time, we discovered that what proved most helpful was a special kind of mental training that involved the cultivation of an open, receptive and non-judgemental acceptance of herself, just as she was at each moment. We focused on her self-criticism and her sense that something was wrong with her – a feeling of some inner flaw that is so common in people who struggle with anxiety. Jennifer worked as hard at her psychotherapy as she had at other aspects of her life, but this therapeutic work didn't involve striving, rushing and, oddly for her, didn't really involve her being 'in control'. Her therapy involved deliberately adopting an attitude of loving kindness towards herself – of being wise and understanding about her anxiety based on what she had learned about how anxiety works. She learned to find her 'inner friend', who offered support and validation in difficult circumstances. From this secure base of self-compassion, she learned how to mindfully pay attention to her present-moment experiences, and to engage in a life of meaning and purpose.

Jennifer had discovered that when she was self-critical, her inner voice was often harsh, angry, and even contemptuous. No friend at all! Having this internal, negatively imbalanced, emotional sense of herself was undermining and significantly increased her experience of stress, anxiety and shame. After all, criticism, whether it is from yourself or another person towards you, is only going to make you feel more stressed out than less so. There is nothing that is soothing, reassuring, encouraging or supportive about self-criticism and one of the most important elements of Jennifer's therapy was the development of her ability to recognize her critical voice as it arose. From here, she was able to learn how to respond to herself with a more supportive, encouraging, warm and compassionate voice. As Jennifer learned, compassion isn't about weakness or some fluffy 'niceness'; it's about how we develop the courage and strength to engage with, and deal with, those things that are difficult for us to do.

This friendly inner voice will in turn help us to pursue our most valued aims and to deal with both our so-called failures *and* our successes.

In time, Jennifer found that the deep reservoir of empathy and care she had reserved for her students was also available for herself. Self-compassion emerged as a powerful presence in her life; she learned to live with occasional feelings of anxiety and to understand that feelings of anxiety are an inevitable, and sometimes valuable, part of life. Through her regular practise of mental training, in and out of her therapy sessions, Jennifer learned to remain calm when in the storm of anxious thoughts and feelings that sometimes moved through her mind and body.

For example, if she had to lead her class in front of the school administrator and an outside evaluator, she would often become physically anxious, and experience tension and shortness of breath before the class began. Her mind would generate all sorts of 'what if?' thoughts and worries such as: 'What if I freeze?' or 'What if I don't seem confident?' But eventually Jennifer learned to divert attention from these thoughts by gently drawing attention to the present moment, by focusing on the flow of her breath going in and out of her body. She learned also to focus some of her attention on the soles of her feet, so that she could feel strong and grounded by her connection to the Earth; thus, she created a new way of 'being with' her anxiety but at the same time engaging in what mattered most to her: being a teacher.

Based upon her training, when anxiety began to arise, Jennifer would take a moment to acknowledge her feelings and then gain perspective on the situation that was unfolding before her. In such times, Jennifer became able to remind herself of the value of her work, and would remind herself of her intention to help her students. If she had to lead her class under an evaluator's close and watchful eye, Jennifer would tell herself: 'Teaching means so very much to me, and I want to do well, and be dedicated to my students and this school. I understand that my mind is on guard against threats, given that I've always found public scrutiny pretty scary, but I know this is just a natural, human response. In this moment, I understand that it's not a fault if I feel some fear, which I can ride as if it were a wave. I can be kind to myself, and do what matters most to me. I'm going to face this situation, and take care of my students.' Jennifer learned to consciously surround herself with warmth, courage and self-acceptance and this deliberate activation of self-compassion awakened an instinctive emotion-regulation system that allows us to feel safe, protected and secure in the presence of a responsive, kind, and nurturing caregiver. This provided Jennifer with just enough emotional space to engage in her lesson, despite her apprehension.

The type of mental training we worked on together is known as Compassionate Mind Training (CMT), and this book aims to bring this training to you. Over these past several years I've worked with many clients like Jennifer, who we shall meet throughout this book, and who were striving intensely to be happy in a highly stressful, competitive environment. A great many of these clients have entered my consultation room and have begun their psychotherapy while suffering from debilitating levels of anxiety, which whispers worries in their minds and creates dreadful imaginary scenarios of nightmarish tomorrows. Such scenarios interrupt their moments of calm and drive up their heart-rates, shorten their breath, alter the rhythm of their breathing and may even make them feel dizzy. As a result, the joys of life, and the simple pleasures of the present moment are all too often swept away in waves of anxiety and negative predictions.

The Experience of Anxiety

The word 'anxiety' comes from the Latin term *anxius*, which means 'a feeling of agitation and upset'. Today, the term anxiety encompasses an array of ways in which we pay attention, feel physically and behave, and these have evolved to help us deal with possible threats in our environment. The first way we might experience anxiety is in the way we feel physically; for example, when you last felt anxious how did it feel to you in your body? What were your physical sensations? Did you have a tingling in your fingers? Or did your stomach tighten? Perhaps your breathing became shallow. Sometimes these physical sensations can themselves make us feel anxious – as if we become anxious about feeling anxious! When that happens people tend to start monitoring how their bodies feel and of course as they do that their anxiety is likely to increase the more they pay attention to it.

If you were to give a one-word label to the emotion that shows up in your mind and in the way you feel physically when you feel anxious, what might it be? 'Fear'? Or, of course, 'anxiety'? Or would you use other words? 'Frustration'? 'Shame'? 'Sadness'? If so, you may understand that our brain translates the physical sensations of anxiety into a complex, uniquely human form of experience that we call emotion. Our five senses blend with memories, stories about ourselves, and our history of thoughts and beliefs to produce an emotional experience in the moment.

Let's imagine that you apply for a job that requires a five-step interview process. During four of these interviews, your potential new bosses look friendly. Each one seems warm and curious; they smile at you, and welcome you into the room; however, the fifth interviewer seems cold and his manner is abrupt. When you look into his eyes they remind you of predatory shark's eyes and you sense hostility. You wonder if he might have several rows of teeth! Well, OK, maybe that is an exaggeration, maybe only two rows – but he really is unnerving! This interviewer looks completely expressionless – flat and hard to read. Which of these interviews would be the one that generates the most tension, and draws more of your attention? Which interview would be most on your mind? Which one would you most likely be brooding over or talking about with your friends at the end of the day?

Similar to Mr Shark Eyes, thoughts or images about things that frighten us are the most distracting and we tend to focus on them more than we focus on thoughts or images that calm us. Additionally, we tend to pay close attention to and remember threats that we have perceived.[1] This means that we have what we call a 'threat-detection system' and it has evolved to be always on, and to operate in a better-safe-than-sorry mode.

When anxiety affects our behaviour it makes us want to do things such as run away or scream. It may make us feel heartbroken, collapse in a protective, tight ball or simply go quiet.

At times, feelings of pain and shame about anxiety may be so great that we may actually wish to die in order to escape. But this book will help you learn how to undermine the pervasiveness of the threat-detection system, and to reclaim your life through compassion and acceptance. Anxiety is one of the most prevalent and challenging forms of human suffering, and it can vary in intensity from mild tension and apprehension to feelings of fear and terror.

During periods of anxiety, our thinking is focused on threats of potential harm and loss, and we can feel an urgent need to run, avoid, freeze or faint. These responses can be triggered very rapidly and often well before we're aware of it happening. We do not choose to have flushes of anxiety – they are part of our physiological make-up that has evolved over millions of years to protect us from possibly harmful situations. Later, we will look at this evolutionary history in greater detail, exploring why it is that we might operate with this always-on threat-detection process humming within us.

Types of Anxiety

It is important to understand that every person has a unique, unfolding relationship with their environment. Our distinct personal histories and our moment-to-moment experiences all interact with and influence our emotions, thoughts and actions. Accordingly, we can notice the differences between us in terms of how anxiety might show up, and also how we might respond to anxious feelings that are unique to and varied in each of us. These variations may relate to what causes us anxiety, how easily our anxiety is triggered, how intense our anxiety is, how frequent it is, the ways we physically and psychologically experience the anxiety, how long the anxiety lasts and correspondingly how easily or quickly we calm down after becoming anxious.

We also know that anxiety takes many different forms. For example, some people can have intense and sudden physical symptoms known as 'panic attacks' that appear to come out of the blue and flush the person with a frightening sense of impending catastrophe. Sometimes this is focused on a physical concern such as fear of having a heart attack. Symptoms such as accelerated heart rate, hyperventilation and catastrophic predictions about death or going insane are common in people who struggle with panic attacks. Other people, however, can suffer from more generalized anxiety, where they experience worries throughout the day about a variety of situations. Generalized anxiety can involve hours lost to immersion in negative predictions. Individuals who feel this way may rarely feel safe, or fully content.

People with social anxiety can become particularly concerned about social situations, fearing that people might see them as inadequate or inferior and, as a consequence, reject or avoid them. Yet other people focus their attention on the way they feel, physically – on their bodily lumps and bumps – constantly worrying about illness and disease. And then there are what we call 'specific phobias', which are anxieties directed to specific things such as the fear of spiders, snakes, heights, and so on. While these categories might seem like neat little boxes within which we can classify different sets of problems, in actuality many of us suffer from more than one of these problems.

Anxiety is an important and essential emotion; however, when people experience levels of anxiety or anxious behaviour that causes significant distress, or impairs their ability to function, they are experiencing what we call an 'anxiety disorder', which negatively affects their lives.

When we look at statistical evidence, we find that people with anxiety disorders are more likely to experience clinical depression[2] and that high levels of anxiety are associated with a range of health problems such as cardiovascular difficulties, high blood pressure, diabetes and chronic fatigue, amongst other medical problems.[3] People who suffer with an anxiety disorder are up to five times more likely to visit their doctor, and up to six times more likely to be hospitalized for psychiatric reasons.[4] If, like so many of us, you have lived with high levels of anxiety, just reading these statistics would probably make you feel even more anxious! But this book will help you understand that anxiety doesn't have to lead to such consequences while at the same time helping you understand how important it is to realize the ways that anxiety can affect our lives.

Think about how high levels of anxiety can affect our relationships; for example, people might have a fear of abandonment and fear of upsetting others and so instead of dealing with conflicts by being honest and open they become submissive, which makes them anxious. The trouble is that the things they are unhappy with don't just go away by themselves, and resentment over feeling submissive, neglected or disempowered, then mixes with anxiety and apprehension, which in turn interferes with the ability to be comfortable in relationships. People with anxiety disorders often experience irritability, are easily distracted, visibly agitated during social interactions, and focus excessively on themselves. Understandably, these sorts of problems also may effect the quality of their relationships.

How Common is Anxiety?

According to the initial findings of the World Health Organization's global mental health survey,[5] anxiety disorders are the most common psychiatric disorder in all but one of the twenty-six countries included in the survey. The initial data from Britain has yet to be reported; however, it is known that nearly 30 per cent of Americans will suffer from an anxiety disorder at some point in their lifetime and it represents nearly 33 per cent of the entire cost of mental-health treatment there,[6] similar to the spending in the UK and in Europe. Considerably more people will suffer from problematic anxiety that might not reach the level of a 'full disorder'.

The vast majority of people with anxiety problems do not come forward for help, partly because they feel ashamed and partly because they feel anxious about the therapeutic process itself: they may be afraid of being prescribed medication; may fear social stigma; or may just be afraid of discussing and facing their fears in the presence of someone else. Other people may not be aware of the existence of effective treatment for anxiety.

2 What is Anxiety and How Has it Evolved?

Many of my clients are pretty clever, and are quick to ask me why anxiety shows up in the ways that it does and how it is that we seem to be programmed to experience it so intensely at times. Hasn't evolution proved that we no longer need this emotion? It's not as if we're living in fear of dinosaurs creeping up on us . . . And why do we still have this emotion as a reaction to those things known to us, things we 'know' to be non-threatening?

When my clients ask if they might be able to get rid of their anxiety altogether, I often ask them what they think would happen if we could totally, miraculously 'zap' their capacity for threat detection out of their minds with some sort of imaginary, science fiction-esque energy beam. If we did this, what would we be left with as an early-warning system of possible threats or dangers? When they thought of it this way, many of my clients realized that, if they didn't have the early-warning system, they would possibly end up being ploughed over by a bus, or a bicycle courier as he weaves his way quietly and at high speed through traffic in order to deliver an urgent message twenty blocks uptown.

For now though, let's imagine our ancestors, those early human cave dwellers out hunting in the jungles. In this situation, a flash of movement in the underbrush might indicate that a vicious predator was about to pounce. This would set their hearts racing as they immediately prepared to flee. Those ancestors who had a sharp enough threat-detection system would be more likely to survive than those who weren't so anxious or afraid, who might then wind up in the belly of a sabre-toothed tiger. Those ancestors who survived would pass their threat-detection genes to their children and so it stands to reason that we wouldn't be here at all if we hadn't emerged from a long line of anxious living beings. But sabre-tooth tigers aren't the only threats to be on the lookout for – we may be injured by falling or by getting into fights or we may become ill by eating or drinking noxious substances. In fact, threats and dangers to our physical and psychological health come in many shapes and sizes and all of those threats need to be detected and dealt with; however, our brain only has one basic system for organizing the bodily processes of threat – not adaptable to each different type of threat. So, this means that whether you are anxious about meeting new people, about being chased down dark alleys by tigers, about losing your wallet on holiday or becoming ill and dying, your basic threat-detection system will stimulate increased anxiety and give you that dreadful bodily sense of anxiety and fear.

Better Safe Than Sorry . . .

Our bodies respond to and deal with threats in our environment similar to the way Customs operates at the airport: nothing much gets through to be processed until the threat system has decided it's safe. This is why your system is so easily aroused, why if you're walking home and hear a sound behind you, you suddenly feel your heart begin to race but then, when you walk a little further and realize you're safe, your threat-detection mode is still on. It needs an outlet, and begins to focus on that lump in your arm that wasn't there yesterday or the possibility that your partner will be in a bad mood when you get home – many different types of small triggers can have big effects inside us. Your threat system is also similar to a factory default setting, in that its first reaction is to be sensitive to possible threats, in all shapes and sizes.

Once the threat-detection system is activated, certain response systems are set in motion. One well known system, which you may have heard of, is the 'fight, flight or freeze' system, whereby our bodies and impulses opt for either a quick escape, aggressive action to protect ourselves, or doing neither and freezing on the spot. We don't choose to do any of these – the way our bodies react is instinctive.

Another defensive strategy is to turn to caregivers for comfort and protection if anxiety or fear arises. Our brains have evolved to make us feel more settled and calmer if we are in the presence of people who care for us and who we think of as protectors. We can see this when we watch how children go to their parents, or their nearest caregivers, for a cuddle when they're upset. Compassion and the kindness of others helps us regulate our inherently trigger-happy threat-response system, which helps regulate our anxiety, and in turn helps us to function in our day-to-day lives. As we will see later, children need the care and affection of their caregivers and friends to help settle down their threat-detection system, as well as teach them how to regulate it themselves and develop their ability to do and confront things that may seem frightening.

Although we might often recognize that our caregivers are crucial to our ability to learn how to cope with anxieties, our friends are also important, particularly as we grow into our teenage years. These people, our caregivers and friends, are called 'attachment figures'. They activate what we call our 'soothing' response and shape our ability to regulate anxiety. We learn from them. In our teens, our friends are likely to be the ones who we will go with to our first parties; they will encourage us to do healthy things, and sometimes dangerous things, as we face new situations and potentially anxiety-inducing social demands.

Our 'affiliation system', which involves our experience of others caring for and about us, is crucial to our ability to respond to anxiety. CFT continually highlights the importance of strengthening the affiliation system from the outside and from within ourselves, and that's why we'll focus on self-compassion-generating exercises later in this book.

I often tell my patients that they were born with an 'Always On, Better-Safe-Than-Sorry Problem-Solving Machine' in their minds. Let's follow this idea in more detail to help us understand why we may feel overwhelmed by anxiety.

Just for a moment, imagine that you are a rabbit chomping on some carrots in a vegetable patch somewhere near your warren. Imagine next that, suddenly, you hear a sound in the bushes or see a flash of movement close by. What is the best thing to do? Is this the time to relax and enjoy the cool breeze on your rabbit fur? No. This is not the time to chill out, bunny style. Nor should you spend too much time thinking about whether what you sensed is, or isn't, a threat. This is the time to assume there is a threat, and to make a break for your rabbit-hole, running (well hopping) as fast as possible. Even if that ominous sound was nothing serious nine times out of ten, or ninety-nine times out of a hundred, it's still better to run, because that sound could have been alerting you, quite literally, to your impending death. One of my colleagues[1] uses a phrase from evolutionary psychology to describe this scenario, and it has stuck with me as a way to remember the importance of our threat-detection system: 'You can skip lunch many times, but you can only be lunch once.'

Have you ever watched birds feeding on a lawn? You will see them peck for a few moments, stop, look around, peck again, stop, look around – and very small sounds and movements will startle them and they will fly away, leaving the food behind. You might think, 'How sad that they don't feel more relaxed and can't just enjoy their meal'; however, as far as we know, the birds aren't feeling sorry for themselves; they are simply working with their 'always-on threat-detection system', and being kept alive with their 'better-safe-than-sorry' behaviour. Who knows when they'll be pounced on by that tabby-cat from next door?

In some contexts, our brains will take very few risks, because of a combination of the 'hardware' of our brain's better-safe-than-sorry threat-detection system, combined with the 'software' of our personal and individual history. We know that we often develop unrealistic estimates of how dangerous the world may be; for example if you asked people to estimate the chances of being burgled or physically attacked they tend to overestimate when they respond.

There is an important implication in this: strange as it may seem, our brains are *designed* to make mistakes, in that they are *designed* to regularly overestimate the possibility of threats. Why? Because doing so increases our chances of survival.

We also know that the threat-detection system can take control of the direction and quality of our attention. Imagine that it's the winter holiday season and that you are shopping for presents. It is crowded and cold, but you are feeling fairly happy, since you are doing something nice for your friends and family. You go to ten shops. In nine shops people are extremely kind and helpful and you've been able to find exactly the right gifts. You come out of each shop feeling pleased; however, in one of the shops the assistant is very rude and unhelpful. You feel irritated and angry with them and leave feeling annoyed and without a present. Which shop assistant do think you'll remember at the end of the day? Which one would you talk about with your partner or friends? Chances are, your attention will focus on the one person who annoyed you rather than the other 90 per cent who were kind and helpful. This is normal – our brains are designed by evolution to focus on and remember the things that are negative, threatening and blocking us. And this is why we need to train our minds to pay attention to the *whole* picture and recognize that sometimes we ignore, or tune out, the positive, helpful things.

Once we become anxious, our minds tend to stay in or return to anxious moments in order to look for confirmation of what we believe to be impending danger. They do this in many ways; for example, your threat-detection system can produce thoughts and images that just pop into your head, even when you are in situations that otherwise appear calm. Sometimes these thoughts might seem strange to us, and we don't understand why they are showing up. For this reason, they are called 'intrusive thoughts'. Imagine, for a moment, that you had an argument with your boss that didn't end perfectly but which was resolved. Isn't it likely that such an argument would be replayed over and over again in your mind? Here is another example: if you watch a horror film you might find disturbing images popping back into your mind even when you don't want them. Those images might make you feel frightened or uneasy, even though you know it's just a film you've seen, and not reality. This aspect of being frightened by our memories and by certain images even when we know they are not accurate shows us that our brain can produce stimuli that make us feel anxious even when we know, rationally, that we should feel calm. This is why sometimes simply relying on rationality doesn't always work. We will come back to this, but my point now is that one of the key features of a well functioning human brain is that it will give priority to focusing on threats and thinking about self-protection, even over and above rationality itself.

It is sometimes said that cognitive therapy (and CFT uses a lot of cognitive techniques) is all about looking at the evidence for and against our negative thoughts, and finding out the truth of our thinking; however, it may not always be helpful or convenient to test the truth of our thinking. It may be more useful or easier to base our behaviour on what works, moment by moment. After all, if you have to escape from the third storey of a burning house via the fire escape it's probably not the most helpful strategy to look down and focus on the fact that, if you fall, you will die.[2] Instead, you should focus on what may help you climb down, or get away, so that you are most likely you survive. So even when our threat-detection system is giving us perfectly accurate information (if you fall, you will die), it's not always the most helpful or compassionate thing to focus on.

Evolution and Forms of Anxiety

In a moment we are going to explore how our bodies and minds can learn to become anxious. There are some fears that evolution has made sure we can acquire very easily, such as the phobia of snakes or spiders rather than the fear of faulty electric light sockets or slippery bathroom floors, even though the fact is that in most countries, certainly in northern Europe and northern American states, you're far more likely to be killed or injured by electricity or by slipping on a wet floor than you are by snakes or spiders. However, electricity and wet floors haven't been around for very long and have not affected our evolution; thus, we need a lot of personal experience to develop a phobia of them. So a fear of snakes or spiders is a common anxiety based on the experiences we've had in the course of our evolution.

Examples of how our current fears relate to threats that our evolutionary ancestors faced

(adapted from Marks & Neese, 1997)

Panic	Threat near alarm and need for help
Fear of snakes/spiders	Difficult to detect and potentially dangerous in our natural ancestral environment
Agoraphobia	Dangerous environment and too distant from a safe base
Claustrophobia	Being trapped in confined spaces and places
Social anxiety	Social put-down and rejection
Paranoia	Group attack or rejection
Hypochondria	Threat to physical health
Compulsive disorder	Avoidance of potential contaminants/illness/disease and also avoidance of spreading disease
Obsessive disorder	Repetitive checking for errors or having done harm
General anxiety	Raised level of awareness in dangerous environments

One of the reasons we like going to the cinema or watching films at home is that the storylines allow us to see and identify with other people who have anxieties and fears and who are facing dangers, and hopefully coping with them; however, observation is also a powerful way to acquire phobias. The psychologists and anxiety experts Michael Cook and Susan Mineka[3] ran a series of experiments in the 1980s that showed one group of monkeys another group of monkeys who were frightened of a toy snake when it was presented to them. The observing group learned to become similarly frightened when toy snakes were introduced to their cage; however, the observing group were also shown another group of monkeys that were reacting fearfully to a flower; however, the observing group showed no fear when the flower was introduced to their own cage. It was thought that perhaps they may have had experiences with other plants and could recognize a flower as harmless. Whatever the precise processes involved, it showed that a monkey's evolutionary history with snakes had likely primed them, and other primates like them such as us humans, to be more likely to acquire a phobia of snakes, even by observation of others acting fearfully, than they might learn to fear something harmless such as a flower.

This is particularly significant in the context of concerns about television and other media that increasingly focus on such things as violence, or on shaming and rejecting people in competitions that throw out a contestant each week, for example. It's unclear what the impact of such programmes is, apart from telling us that we are constantly being judged and can easily be found wanting. This is unfortunate, given that the fear of social rejection is a major social anxiety for humans because our survival has depended upon acceptance and sharing, and given also that our fears are often shaped and easily developed by our current social environment.

Remember Jennifer and her first panic attack in the subway? Well, entrapment (claustrophobia) is a natural danger to humans and if we are in a state of anxiety, tired or stressed, our brains tend to flick through our files of potential dangers, spot one and then set off the alarm. This sounds like what may have happened with Jennifer, who was already in an anxious state and whose brain likened the experience of being in a closed subway carriage to being trapped, and as a result it pushed the alarm button. This is why she found relief when she went out into the fresh air. In fact, it is common for people to become claustrophobic if they are already slightly anxious. In some ways what's more extraordinary is the fact that people in their millions go to work on trains and subways often crushed together!

But just as we can learn that something is dangerous, we can also learn that some things that trigger our threat-detection system don't need to trigger our alarms. This is fundamental to our understanding of how we can regulate our senses and regulate our threat-response system: if you have experienced a high degree of anxiety in a certain situation, it is likely that being in that situation again, or even being in a *similar* situation, will trigger your response, your 'threat-response'. If I suffered an embarrassing failure in delivering a speech about ancient history when I was a small child, I still may quiver a bit when I have to stand before a group of colleagues and speak about sales figures, for example.

To really understand how we learn our patterns of response to anxiety, we need to look at how we and other animals learn from our interactions with our environments.

Anxiety Learned by Association

So far, a great deal of what we've discussed has been about the way we have evolved to be able to react and deal with threats in our environment; however, we have also evolved to easily acquire feelings of anxiety and physical and mental responses to those feelings.

Behavioural scientists often describe two basic learning processes that contribute to the way we learn to respond to situations. The first is often called Classical Conditioning and was discovered by Russian physiologist, Ivan Pavlov (1849–1936), who became interested in how our stomachs respond to food, or the promise of food. It was well known that the smell of food could make dogs salivate; what Pavlov discovered was that if he regularly sounded a bell before giving the dogs their dinner, the dogs would begin to salivate at the sound, regardless of whether food was produced afterwards or not. Normally, the ringing bell would not make an animal salivate but these dogs had *acquired* that physical response (salivating) because of an *association* (the sound of the bell signalling that food would be dished out).

Classical Conditioning, or learning by association, has become important to our understanding of anxiety because we have found that our threat-response systems respond not only to the sound of the bell, but also to sounds that are similar. This is called 'generalization', or 'discrimination' learning. And the sound of the bell may not just be an indication of positive things such as food or treats; it could also be an indication, or a warning, of negative things. Suppose that every time a bell was rung, Pavlov's dog was given a mild electric shock. The dog would then develop a cowering fear of the bell ringing, rather than a tail-wagging, salivating, 'where's my food?' response. This fearful response to the ringing of the bell is known as 'aversive' conditioning, but it is still learning by association. And from this we can see that the bell can acquire any kind of physiological effect depending upon what it is paired, or associated, with and this means that almost any neutral stimulus, such as a bell, can create physiological reactions in us because of what we've linked it with, or what it's been linked to, previously. Likewise, if you've felt anxious because of something in the past, you will associate this certain something, be it giving a speech or a hairy spider or a crowded train, with anxiety in the future. Your brain and response system have learned that this will make you anxious, and react accordingly.

Here's a different scenario: let's imagine that when I was a little boy my house was burgled in the middle of the night when I was at home. Hearing the smashing glass of the window and sensing the hurried, purposeful rumbling movement of a team of criminals would suddenly provoke in me a feeling of fear, and a desire to get to safety. That would be automatic, and in such a situation I might learn to associate some of the other elements of the environment, such as the time of night, the furniture in the room, or the ticking of the clock with this moment of danger and terror. Later in life, my fear from that situation might generalize to anxiety when I went to bed or to a startled response to noises outside of my bedroom. As a result, I might fear going back to bed; thus, as a result of this burglary I learned, or was 'conditioned', to fear my bedroom because what I felt when I was there (fear) is something I associate with the burglary. An otherwise neutral element of my environment (a bedroom) has become associated with a frightening event (a burglary).

OK. So now we know that anxiety can be triggered because of what we've learned in the past. But we should also understand that anxiety can be triggered without any learning at all, and includes our responses to things such as sudden loud noises, aggressive, threatening people, large open spaces, animals coming towards us, heights and so on – our basic anxiety responses can be associated with all kinds of things. Let's look at another example: imagine a child, let's call him Fred, whose father was aggressive and who, if Fred had made him angry, would send him to his room to wait; then eventually, Fred's dad would enter the room, scream at him and beat him. Understandably, Fred used to be very anxious when he waited in his room, which was decorated with a particular type of wallpaper. Fred grew up and had forgotten about this until one day he went to see a new doctor for a check-up. He walked into the surgery and the doctor smiled at him but Fred immediately began to feel overwhelming anxiety. Not knowing what was happening to him was very alarming and disorientating; however, after a few moments, it dawned on him that the wallpaper in the doctor's surgery was similar to the wallpaper in his boyhood room. Through associative learning and Classical Conditioning, Fred's body remembered how he felt when he was a child and this memory helped to recreate his physical and mental feelings of anxiety.

This 'body memory' as we now call it, can be somewhat controversial because it is sometimes used to support theories about repressed memories. In CFT we aren't really concerned with these, and when we use the term 'body memory', we simply mean the way that our nervous system via our physical body and our mental functioning – our brain – can evoke a response that we have learned and which we then physically feel. It can be triggered by any of our five senses: sight, hearing, taste, smell, touch.

Here is another example. Imagine going to a party where you have a pint of beer or a piece of cake but within a little while you feel quite ill and not long after you are vomiting violently. Eventually you recover and after a few weeks you've forgotten about it. You go to another party but as you step through the door somebody gives you a pint of beer or a piece of cake. What do you think happens to your body? Just the smell of the beer or the sight of the cake could give you a flash of nausea. Your body remembers immediately and rapidly. Suppose, however, you'd forgotten about the party where you'd become sick or suppose Fred had forgotten about the association of the wallpaper in the room where he was beaten.

The problem is that, even if you may think you'd forgotten, your body will remember, so what you're left with is a physiological (physio = body; logical = mind) flash of anxiety or nausea that you might not be able to fully understand.

A part of our brain called the amygdala is responsible for body memory and it is active from birth; the part of our brain that allows us to remember time and place, to remember when and where bad things happen to us is called the hippocampus, but this matures and becomes active much later. Some researchers think that we can acquire body-memory anxieties before we can accurately locate them in time and place and that this could be a reason why some people experience certain types of anxiety that they can't identify the cause of, or any specific reason for. In CFT we aim to develop a healthy response to our anxiety through new emotional experiences that directly influence and affect how the amygdala works.

There is one other aspect to anxiety and conditioning that affects us and this is the fact that we can become affected by, and respond to, not only things in the outside world but also those things inside us. Many years ago, a behavioural psychologist[4] noted that if children are constantly punished for being angry they will become anxious about being punished and over time their feelings of anger will become associated with the expectation of punishment and the expectation of punishment activates anxiety. After a while, the system or cycle short-circuits; thus, the feelings of anger automatically trigger feelings of anxiety. What happens then is that when conflicts arise, instead of feeling anger and learning to be assertive, the person simply becomes overwhelmed with anxiety about their own potential anger. There are many therapies that suggest that sometimes anxiety is driven by a person's inability to deal with other emotions, including anger. So if you suffer from anxiety it's always worth thinking about how you deal with conflicts and how comfortable you are with your anger.

There are other internal 'things' that can become associated with anxiety. For example, sexual fantasies and sexual feelings are also common sources of anxiety. If you are homosexual but live in a place that is extremely hostile towards homosexuality, you may become anxious about your feelings and desires. As soon as they pop into your mind you might begin to have anxiety attacks. Or if you live somewhere that is extremely conservative you may experience anxiety about your own liberal sexual views and beliefs, which seem to be in contrast to the status quo.

We will come back to the fear of such internal things later. For now, it is important to note the fact that sometimes we can have automatically anxious responses without realizing the emotions sitting behind them.

Anxiety Learned by Consequences

So the first type of learning we've explored is called Classical Conditioning, or learning by association, and it relates to the way our brains and bodies automatically respond to certain triggers, and how some new things in our environment can become associated with these triggers and evoke a response similar to the one we experienced originally.

The second type of learning is based on how the consequences that follow our actions influence the degree to which we repeat a behaviour. This second type helps us find out what kind of learning might lead to the increase or decrease of a behaviour on the basis of consequences such as rewards and punishments. (This type of learning can be called 'Operant Conditioning'; however, that term never really had a ring to it for me, as it sort of wades out into some pretty technical language and I think that, for our purposes, we can think of it simply as 'learning from consequences'.)

Put plainly, if we repeatedly experience a pleasant or desirable consequence after we behave in a certain way, we are more likely to repeat that behaviour. Also, if we experience an unpleasant or painful consequence after a behaving in a certain way, we are less likely to behave that way again, or as frequently. For example, if a child completes their homework on time, and is then praised by her parents, who give her a 'bonus' in her weekly allowance, this reward might contribute to more frequent, timely homework-completion behaviour. Similarly, if a child returns home after their curfew, and is punished by not being allowed to play any video games for a weekend, this punishment may reduce this curfew-breaking behaviour in the future. Now, we all know that learning, and particularly parenting, isn't quite that simple, but these are the basic principles that allow people to learn to behave in a certain way after repeated experiences of reward or punishment for that behaviour.

When it comes to the dynamics of learning, anxiety can seem very tricky. Both the learning processes we've looked at contribute to our ability to learn to re-experience anxiety over the course of our lives. If we look at the example of a fear of social situations, we can begin to see how what we call 'learning theory' (the scientific theory about learning) might shed a little more light on how anxiety operates. More importantly, we can get a sense of how our best efforts to avoid anxiety can actually make it worse.

Let's imagine that Jennifer, who we met earlier, had been a bookish, reserved yet friendly teenager. Imagine that perhaps one day she went to a school dance and was filled with hopes to be popular, make friends, or just feel approved of by a group of her buddies. She wore her best outfit, and tried to be 'cool'. At the dance some other teenage girls, who were hungry to assert their own place at the top of the high-school popularity food chain, decided to bully and tease her. They joked about her being a 'geek', and laughed at her as she danced. Because of this experience, Jennifer later began to associate social events with being mocked. This is an example of Classical Conditioning, which trained her to feel fear, experience self-doubt and expect to be bullied when she approaches social situations.

How might Jennifer respond to invitations for social events, and gatherings of people in the future? Well, we've seen that we have evolved with an 'always on, better-safe-than-sorry' threat-detection system that helps us to steer clear of danger, yes? And in this case Jennifer's threat-detection system responds by avoiding social situations that provoke anxiety. With this avoidance, we can see the beginning of learning by consequences, which builds on the foundation of Classical Conditioning, or learning by association. And these together help establish and then maintain Jennifer's anxiety.

By avoiding a social event, Jennifer relieves her anxiety and releases any tension in the immediate short term. That release actually rewards and then reinforces her behaviour, which she will then repeat. And the cycle continues. In this case, her behaviour is worrying about, and becoming anxious about, going to a party. Paradoxically, her avoidance is actually training her to feel more anxiety in the long term: by avoiding social experiences, Jennifer is consistently teaching herself to remain afraid of contact with other people; however, this is not the end of the story because one of the key points of CFT is that it often depends upon the degree of helpfulness and kindness we have around us when we experience these kinds of event. We know for example that anxious parents tend to increase the anxiety in their children because if their children have been bullied, for example, the parents will encourage their children to avoid subsequent social situations where they may be bullied again. To them it makes common sense: why would they want to see their child so unhappy? Why would they encourage them back into those situations that are obviously unpleasant? Why? To learn to confront the bullies or any other difficult situation, and to learn how to deal with the situation better than if it were avoided altogether, to learn to be assertive, how to find other friends, how to cope with their feelings, even if they may be unpleasant. We learn nothing from avoidance other than avoidance, which may reinforce the experience of anxiety itself and may make us critical of ourselves for our behaviour, and then feel unhappy about missing out, which is typical of children who feel bullied. Some people even begin to dislike themselves for the thing they are bullied about, whether it be shyness or being overweight or a bit clumsy. So how is that child going to overcome or learn to work on their anxiety when they are also self-critical?

But if you were Jennifer's friends, or her parents who weren't anxious, what would you do? Would you encourage her to avoid a similar situation? Would you be critical and force her to go out? Or would you be understanding and compassionate, but also encouraging and support-ive, step by step, to help develop her confidence? The chances are that you would do the latter and that's key to understanding the steps in CFT. You see? You already have the inner wisdom of how to deal with your anxiety because when you think about an example like this you probably know exactly what to do; however, when it comes to your own anxiety you may well have critical thoughts about it, try to avoid or suppress it or feel ashamed of it, rather than feel kind, supportive, encouraging and understanding towards yourself, as you would towards Jennifer.

So, even though we have intuitive wisdom to be compassionate we can still fall back into a spiral of anxiety and avoidance, which is sometimes called 'safety behaviour' and which can lead to an amplification of our response to anxiety, and to an increase in our suffering. It seems that the more we try to avoid, change or suppress our experiences of anxiety, the more the anxiety is intensified in the long term. Psychological research has revealed that our best attempts to stifle or push away thoughts and feelings often backfire.[5]

In a classic example, let's imagine that you agree to take part in a psych-ology experiment at university, and that you are given a simple set of instructions: for the next five minutes, don't think of a purple gorilla. Every time you think of that purple gorilla, make a check mark on this piece of paper in front of you. How many check marks might you make? For most people, it will be a heck of a lot. When we try not to think of that gorilla, there he is again, dancing the lavender simian cha-cha. The reason suppression operates like this is straightforward – you have to keep checking that you're suppressing your thoughts – and in order to do this you have to keep revisiting what you're trying to suppress just to make sure nothing creeps out around the edges. And because you've associated *not* suppressing with something that is frightening your fear system will keep pushing you to remember it.

Beyond what we've learned so far, it's important to recognize that every time you think, 'Don't think of a purple gorilla,' you have just thought of a purple gorilla. Similarly, if you are telling yourself, 'Don't think anxiety-provoking thoughts,' you are thinking anxiety-provoking thoughts.

However, what happens if we turn the experiment on its head? In our contrasting experiment the instructions are simply: observe whatever thoughts you might have, and feel free to think anything at all. If you happen to think about a purple gorilla, please make a check mark on this piece of paper. The meandering nature of mental activity would likely wander through all sorts of topics. From time to time that purple gorilla might pop up in your imagination. It is, after all, a rather odd instruction. We can reliably predict, though, that you won't be making as many check marks when you allow your mind to just be where it is. That gorilla doesn't show up as often if we aren't actively wrapped up in trying to push his image away.

Part of our training in developing self-compassion and mindful awareness will involve changing our relationship to our experiences and this is not done by struggling with and avoiding emotions such as anxiety. Self-compassion and loving kindness allow us to develop an openness to our present-moment experiences and to then remain connected to difficult feelings, and to develop new ways of responding to those things that scare us. In this way, we can witness our own pain and fear, and develop the ability to respond with kindness, patience and effective action.

Traditional behaviour therapy trains people to remain in the presence of those things that trigger anxiety until the anxiety response has run its course. For example, if I were afraid of heights my behavioural therapist might take me, one step at a time, to a window on a very high floor of a tall building. I would edge closer to the window, staying with each step until the anxiety decreases, and then I would take another step. This is called 'exposure' as I am slowly teaching my body that everything is actually OK. Because I do not act on my fears, my response system gradually settles down. The lesson will be anxiety-provoking at first, but if I remain in the presence of what I fear, or what triggers my fear, without avoiding it, my anxiety is likely to gradually decrease. In time, with repeated learning experiences, I will be able to respond differently and without fear or avoidance. This type of therapy is often referred to as 'exposure', and it has been proven to be effective for treating problems with anxiety.

Exposure with Compassion

While exposure has a good track record in the treatment of anxiety, CFT goes beyond this method, and seeks to do more than just train people to exhaust their anxiety responses. Imagine that you are in therapy to deal with the anxiety caused by your fear of heights. Imagine on the one hand that your therapist seems competent, very understanding, patient, caring, smiles at you and encourages you. You feel safe with your therapist. On the other hand, imagine that your therapist seems competent but is also standoffish, doesn't smile very much, tells you what to do but doesn't particularly encourage you or seem friendly towards you. Which therapist do you want and which do you think you can have most success with? Not a difficult question is it? Likewise, we are more able to engage with things that frighten us if we are in a supportive environment. Children in particular can engage with things that are frightening if those people who they trust are around them to encourage them and give them friendly signals. A lovely example of this can be seen in what has been called the 'Visual Cliff Experiments', which you can see for yourself at: www.youtube.com/watch?v=eyxMq11xWzM&feature=related.

CFT points out that just as the experience of understanding, kindness, encouragement and genuine feelings of being cared about will help us engage in things that are difficult, so too will developing this attitude and emotional tone to ourselves be immensely helpful. When they first come to see me, many of my clients lack this inner compassionate tone directed towards themselves and, if anything, dislike themselves for being anxious, which they often think of as a weakness or inadequacy. At the very least, they are hostile to their anxiety. As we will see, training ourselves to be self-compassionate activates an innate emotion-regulation system, which involves a deep appreciation of suffering, and a loving aspiration to alleviate that suffering. It stems from the same evolutionary source as a mother's care and attention towards her young. When we have self-compassion we can remain in the presence of difficult feelings, with a wide, accepting, flexible awareness and as a result we can learn new, workable and engaging ways of responding to even the most challenging and anxiety-provoking situations, thoughts and sensations.

3 Anxiety, Compassion and Our Ongoing Interactions with the World

We can see how millions of years of evolution coupled with our unique personal histories can make us particularly sensitized to anxious feelings, and that this can lead to 'trouble'. There is no doubt about it though: our anxiety can save our lives. Our awareness of danger can keep our physical bodies safe; however, anxiety can save us in non-physical ways, too, can't it? Yes, it can, by alerting us to all sorts of things that we need to pay attention to in our personal, professional and academic lives. For example, if we become anxious before an exam we may make some special efforts to ensure we prepare as best as we can. Similarly, feeling a little bit extra aware of danger on the highway might mean that we pay closer attention to our driving. You might be anxious if you feared your child was ill, and this might make you ring for the doctor just that much sooner. Anxiety is basically a system designed by evolution to help us and to guide us towards actions that may protect us. So far so good, except that it doesn't always work quite so smoothly, and when it doesn't it can be a real hassle and cause all sorts of distress.

Enduring a hair-triggered threat-detection system is like having smoke detectors that keep going off when there's even a hint of warm air. When our anxiety thresholds are chronically raised, which can happen when we live in stressful environments, our anxiety can become an unwelcome guest. It's still part of our basic protection system, but now it's showing up when we don't need it to and will feel too intense, and can last too long.

In order to understand our anxiety response, and eventually reach a place of safety and calm, even when our fears are triggered, it will help to recognize that anxiety emerges through some important interactions between us and our environment. Our personal history can contribute to how and why we feel anxious, just as our genetic history has contributed to our capacity for threat detection. The particular stressful situations that we face in our everyday lives are also factors that can lead to our anxiety levels feeling problematic. Our moods, our relationships and many other aspects of our lives can help trigger our threat-detection system in ways that don't really help us, and which contribute to our suffering.

When I think of my client Jennifer, whom we met in the first chapter, I remember the many elements that came together for her that day on the subway to create a perfect storm that led to her panic attack. Let's look at a few of these factors to help us understand just how anxiety problems can manifest themselves:

The day that she first called me, Jennifer was facing a great deal of stress in the form of strict new evaluation programmes that had been put in place in her school system that year. Her new term was about to begin, and she desperately wanted to live up to the relentlessly high standards of the administration. The engine of her mind kept churning away about this, seeking new ways to ensure that she would be perceived as 'above average' or even, gasp, 'superior'.

On top of this, a few weeks earlier, her boyfriend of many years had told her that he needed to 'take a break' from their relationship and explained that he would prefer to date other people, for a while at least. This was very sad for her, as she was really devoted to him, and had secretly planned that they would wind up married and living happily ever after. She hadn't, however, allowed herself to tell him about this plan.

Beyond this, Jennifer had been raised by parents who were completely wrapped up in the idea of success and achievement and who focused much of their efforts on pushing her to be in complete control of her emotions. They were involved, supportive and caring parents in principle but their beliefs about emotional control and achievement eclipsed their ability to nurture, accept and soothe their children. In Jennifer's family, effectiveness, conscientiousness and academic excellence were prized above emotional expression, uncertainty and spontaneity. Any hint that she was feeling out of control led Jennifer to suspect that there was something fundamentally damaged, flawed and unlovable about her. In turn, she relied on avoidance-based coping strategies, such as avoiding social contact, restricting her expressions of emotion, and attempting to suppress thoughts and emotions, all of which trained her to feel more and more anxiety in a range of different situations.

Much later in her therapy, Jennifer tearfully admitted that she always suspected that she would eventually lose her mind and die alone in a psychiatric hospital. She believed this because she had been taught that her emotions amounted to weakness and if uncontrolled would lead to insanity. No one had explained to her, or understood themselves, that anxiety was a natural part of being alive, or that anxious feelings would rise and fall like waves, as do all mental experiences. As Jennifer and I worked together, we gradually unpacked the way these different threads of her life had interwoven and created a response system that was entirely preoccupied with threat detection. As a result, anxiety and a very real terror around the basic act of living were virtually destined to dominate her experiences: she constantly felt fearful and ashamed. We can see though that Jennifer's anxiety and her way of trying to deal with it was not her fault.

If we stand back and recognize that our brains are built to generate powerful emotions, we can also stand back to realize that our experience of these emotions is absolutely not our fault. Moreover, if early in life we don't learn what our emotions and internal responses mean, or learn healthy and functional ways to deal with them, our inner lives can become particularly problematic. Again, it is important to know that this is no fault of our own.

Perhaps now would be a good time to pause, spend a minute, maybe close your eyes, and focus on the fact that your anxiety is not your fault. Slowly, kindly and gently say this over and over again to yourself, whether out loud or in your mind. Note any resistance, any other voices that say, 'Yes, but . . .'

Understand that your mind has been constructed to feel anxiety and that certain events or experiences in your life have in some way activated the system in you. If you begin to develop a non-critical, kind and understanding voice, you are taking the first steps towards a compassionate approach to your anxiety. Don't worry if this seems more difficult than it sounds; it is common for people to struggle with being kind to themselves and to stop blaming themselves for their anxiety.

If you think about Jennifer's story it may become clearer: her pain was not her fault. And if you understand this to be true for her, then perhaps you can see it applying to you. In this moment, as you read this book on compassion and anxiety, allow yourself to hold on to this idea lightly, even for a few moments: 'It is not my fault.' This step and this recognition will help you begin your journey to self-compassion, into letting go of shame and blame.

You did not choose to have a brain that is capable of intense anxiety, nor did you choose to have anxiety difficulties; they really are not your fault. However, you can learn to be honest about them, change your relationship with them and live with them in conditions of greater ease.

Anxiety, Compassion and 'The Man with Two Brains'

'The Man with Two Brains' or 'The Woman with Two Brains' would be a great title for a science-fiction movie, wouldn't it? Come to think of it, the comedian and actor Steve Martin starred in a film in the 1980s with that title already, so I guess copyright laws need to be respected. We can't use it for a movie title, but we can use the idea of having two brains to understand that, in fact, we have a number of 'different' brains that we can look at from the top to the bottom or even from left to right or back to front, because different areas of the brain are responsible for different functions of our behaviour. We like to think that the functions of the brain always work as a team – and often they do – but sometimes different functions within our brain can conflict with one another. What I want to bring to your attention is the fact that our brains are formed so that they are roughly divided into two regions that represent different stages of evolution.

Of course, this is an oversimplification; a neuroscientist, or even a ten-year-old with access to a computer can show you full colour, 3D representations of a whole host of different brain regions, each one involved in different parts of the way we function; however, it is useful to notice two distinct aspects of the brain: the 'old brain' and the 'new brain'. For many years neuroscientists have been pointing to the importance of distinguishing between motivation systems and emotional systems and the more recently evolved systems that enable us to think and have a sense of self.

A simple way of thinking about this is that there are parts of our brain that we can trace back hundreds of millions of years and other parts of the brain that are much more recent. Some scientists talk about how the oldest parts of the brain have been involved with the four F's: feeding, fighting fleeing and . . . reproduction; however, when we mammals evolved our brains developed to make us able to care for our infants. And much later when we humans evolved we developed so that we were capable of thinking for ourselves and imagining the future and so on. And it is useful to make a rough distinction between the old brain, which we share with many other mammals and which is concerned with our basic emotions such as anxiety, anger, joy, sexual interest and motives, forming friendships, belonging to groups, and our new brain, which gives us the capacity for reasoning and thinking.

CFT uses this understanding of the different parts of the brain, albeit in a simplified way, to help us make sense of the complicated link between thinking and the systems in our bodies that produce often very strong physical and impulsive urges. And, again, these are our 'factory default settings'. Indeed, one of the important aspects of CFT is the consideration of how old and new brain systems interact. Obviously, humans have a uniquely large capacity for language, imagination, planning and conceptualization that we don't share with even our most complex and intelligent animal relatives. We can imagine the future and worry about it; remember and fret about the past; and wonder about how we are thought of by others. We can develop sophisticated verbal theories about who in our office likes us, who has it in for us, and what their specific reasons for their opinions might be. All of this winds up expanding the number of things we can feel anxious about and increases the likelihood of holding anxiety in our minds.

Animal mental activity is very different; for example, no matter how clever they may be, monkeys don't sit in trees taking their pulse, and they don't look at their reflections and worry about putting on too much weight or going bald. Zebras don't stay up at night worrying about where the lions will be in the morning, and they certainly don't worry about the careers of their children.

The distinctive nature of our human experience has to do with our fantastically evolved, blindingly efficient 'new brain'; however the structures this rests upon and interacts with are parts of our brain that are 'older', in evolutionary terms. And in order to understand anxiety, compassion and our emotional lives, it helps to understand this 'old brain' and how it functions.

The philosopher Alan Watts once emphasized that 'We don't come into the world, we come out of it.' The entire spectrum of our motivations, emotions, aspirations, and mental capacities has emerged from a complex, ongoing process of evolution, which allows us to trace the genetic and historical roots of our inner and outer behaviours. The brain systems that are involved with some of our most basic emotions such as anger, fear or disgust are millions of years older than our species[1] and, as we touched on earlier, animals have been functioning in 'fight, flight or freeze mode' to survive and protect themselves for a very long time. Our brain structures and nervous-system interactions that support these protection emotions and behaviours are similar to those we might have found in earlier mammals, and even in reptiles. These structures and interactions are what we are referring to when we speak about the 'old brain'.

Studies of chimpanzees who are engaged in the pursuit of sexual and social relationships show that: they strive for dominance and status in their own social hierarchies and that they are capable of looking after one another. They communicate with each other and ask for help or protection in times of danger and need. Chimpanzees team up to hunt, and seek comfort in one another's company when they are frightened. Apart from chimps, other animals such as the simple crow, which happens to be a very clever bird, can roughly deduce the intentions of other animals in their environment. They call to one another to warn of danger, and either compete for or share their resources.[2] A great many of the emotions, motives, and social behaviours that we think of as fundamentally human have actually been present in other species far longer than we have been renting space on this planet. Some of the most prominent features of old-brain emotions are anger, anxiety, sadness, joy and lust; old-brain behaviours include responses of fight, flight, withdrawal or direct engagement with another organism or situation. In the realm of relationships we can see features such as the pursuit of sex, power, status, tribalism, and attachment behaviours towards others.

In addition to these, we have a wide range of capacities that are related to our 'new brain', some of which set us apart from other animals. In particular, we humans have a region of the new brain that is involved in a host of activities that are distinctly ours and which is unique in its power, structure and function. It is called our 'prefrontal cortex'. A lot of these new-brain capacities have to do with language, thinking, imagination, planning, and problem solving.

Our new brain allows us to be uniquely capable of crafting symbolic mental and verbal representations of our environment and ourselves. We can understand the world around us by making a simple observation such as 'that rock looks bigger than the other rock' or by something more complex such as theoretical calculus or the poetic wordplay of Shakespeare. One of the miracles of human new-brain capacity is that we can learn through conditioning and through the consequences of our actions, but also through observation, deduction, and indirect experience. We also have an amazing ability to be self-aware, which allows us to observe even our own acts of observation.

Overall, the new brain allows us the ability to imagine, plan, think and communicate by using our written and spoken language and also to construe our sense of self, and our self-awareness.

How does this relate to anxiety? Well, part of the problem with anxiety involves the collision of old-brain emotions and purposes with the fascinating capacities of our new brain. Let's return to the example of Jennifer to look at how her two brains might be interacting when she struggles with anxiety.

Jennifer's old brain has set her up to respond to any perceived threat with a rapid fight, flight or freeze response, based on the 'always on, better-safe-than-sorry' principle. Her old brain has evolved to seek status, approval of the group, attachment to others, fear of being shunned in social interactions and to avoid getting trapped in potentially dangerous environments. We have seen that her history has emphasized and reinforced the act of seeking acceptance, the expectation of rejection in social situations and that as a result she has been conditioned to have an anxiety response in a situation that might involve social evaluation. We've also seen the threat to her romantic attachment, and such a threat can also raise our anxiety threshold, as it has done so with her. It is common for people who have experienced separations or major losses to experience increased anxiety, and this is another example of the interaction between anxiety and our sense of safety created through our secure and compassionate relationships. All of this – the motivations, the learned behaviour and the emotions – can be thought of as originating in the old brain.

But it doesn't stop there. Jennifer is bright, and she has lots of finely honed new-brain capacities such as self-awareness. While lying awake at night, the stirrings of her old brain interact with her new brain, and take the form of a stream of worrisome predictions about how the rest of her life will unfold. If we remind ourselves of Jennifer's early history and some of the events in her recent life we can notice how she had become much more inwardly self-focused. She would tell herself: 'I'm going to be like this forever, I know it. Everyone at school can see I'm a nervous wreck and there's just no way out. I'm a fraud. I try to seem so competent, but I'm barely functioning. Who would want to be with a person like this? No wonder my boyfriend's left me. I'm going to die alone after living in a squalid apartment with thirty cats!' And while she is thinking about this, her new brain is unspooling corresponding images. She would see herself being scowled at, and almost smell the dank apartment where she imagines she will grow old, all alone. Her new brain has a necessary tendency to respond to imaginary things as if they were real, and this means that her heart would pound, her stomach churn, and her body and mind prepare themselves for what they perceive to be a life-threatening situation, despite the fact that she would be lying safely in bed, miles away from such an experience. But her old brain tends to narrow and focus her attention to help her avoid potential danger, whether it is real or imagined. And when she then tries to suppress potentially distressing thoughts and feelings, her efforts backfire and instead keep her focused on her recurring anxieties. From this scenario, we can see how old-brain activity can mingle with new-brain abilities to stir up our anxiety.

4 Towards the Compassionate Mind: An Evolution in Our Understanding of Anxiety through Mindfulness, Acceptance and Compassion

'Talk therapy' and psychiatric medication are relatively recent developments that took shape during the last century; however, we have been devising clever ways of coping with anxiety and other difficult emotions since the earliest days of civilization.

Opiates were used to alter states of consciousness and to communicate with the gods in rituals as early as 3,400 BC.[1] Throughout history and in cultures the world over, shamans, mystics and tribal leaders have been consulted when people faced emotional problems or needed guidance. Sometimes the consultations occurred in face-to-face meetings or rituals, when herbal 'medicine' might have been prescribed. In India, as much as 3,000 years ago, there is evidence that methods of meditation and yoga were developed to calm and centre the mind in response to anxiety and other troubling emotions.[2]

In his seminal work *The Observing Self*, Arthur Deikman traces the tradition of psychotherapy back through what he sees as its historical roots[3] and suggests that the work modern psychotherapists engage in descends from centuries of meetings between priests, mystics and people who felt troubled, and wanted to talk about their problems. Until the industrial revolution, these efforts to work through difficult emotions and problems had a spiritual or pre-scientific rationale but as our scientific understanding of the brain, mind and behaviour has evolved, so have our theories about anxiety, and our methods for treatment.

With the advent of more traditional psychotherapy over the past 120 years or so, there have been a range of new ideas about the causes of anxiety. In turn, these new ideas have brought about new suggestions for how to deal with it. Although much of their work is based on the science of learning, behaviourists such as Ivan Pavlov, who we mentioned earlier, have also suggested that some of our fears are inherited and due to our biological make-up. Others, such as Pavlov's contemporary, the groundbreaking psychotherapist Sigmund Freud, believed that our behaviour was the result of the suppressed wishes and desires that we harbour in our subconscious. Years later, in the late 1960s and early 1970s, rapidly advancing computer technology and advances in research about cognition and perception led to what is now known as the 'Cognitive Revolution' in psychology: rather than focusing on supposedly subconscious desires, or looking at models of animal behaviour, psychotherapists became increasingly interested in how humans process information. Based on the work of Aaron T. Beck and Albert Ellis, schools of 'cognitive therapy' emerged[4] and promoted the idea that it's often our interpretations of reality, patterns of thinking, and negative biases that lead to problems with anxiety.

According to a cognitive therapist, if someone has a rush of anxiety and feels their heart racing they will panic only if they also have the thought that maybe they could lose control or have a heart attack. The process that takes the anxiety to a problematic level, according to cognitive therapists, is the negative automatic thoughts that we have about perceived threats. We know that people naturally feel somewhat socially anxious when meeting new people or socializing (this is why alcohol is so commonly consumed at parties) and of course some people are shyer than others. Cognitive theory suggests that anxiety becomes problematic when people start to buy into the perception that others see them as inferior, inadequate, boring or stupid (for example). Many of us also have various anxieties about our physical health – after all, none of us wants to become ill, be incapacitated or die. However, few of us suffer from such health-related anxiety; rather, for most of us, worries about health come and go without us being overly focused on them. But people with hypochondriacal anxieties have frequent, intense thoughts that they could be ill, even if they have just emerged from the GP surgery with a clean bill of health. They might tell themselves that the doctors are miss-ing something and this leads them to seek reassurance repeatedly, which only works for a while, as they go back to thinking, 'Maybe the doctors have missed something or maybe something has changed between the time I visited the doctor and now.'

Another side effect of anxiety is vivid imagination; for example, people who have problems with panic can have clear visions or mental images of themselves keeling over and collapsing; people who have social anxiety might have images of other people ridiculing them and secretly wanting to distance themselves.

The cognitive-therapy approach focuses on the meanings that we give to different triggers and experiences and seeks to help people overcome anxiety by noticing anxiety-stimulating thoughts, and directly changing such thinking in order to reduce distress. This can happen through a systematic questioning of negative, automatic thoughts and which takes place in therapy sessions, and by using homework exercises.

All these approaches have some merit; however, good science always moves on in an effort to improve understanding and the effectiveness of interventions. Over the past decade, a quiet revolution has taken place in the sciences of the mind and psychotherapy. Eastern mind-training traditions and Western psychology have come together in an unprec-edented fashion, allowing the development of new psychotherapies that build on and add to our understanding of anxiety and how to cope with it. Concepts such as mindfulness, acceptance, compassion and self-compassion that were once solely associated with Eastern meditative practices or dismissed as 'new-age' are now central therapeutic concepts and the subject of worldwide research.

Many of these approaches focus on the ability of anxiety to easily grab our attention and hold it firmly in its grasp. Mindfulness and acceptance-based psychotherapies point out that, with patience and awareness, we can choose what we pay attention to, or attend to, moment by moment. We can also learn to pay attention to aspects of our mind that are specifi-cally designed to regulate and calm down our threat-detection systems:

just as a child anxiously runs back to his or her mother for a calming, loving embrace, so too can we direct our attention to inner images that evoke feelings of kindness, understanding and support for a calming and soothing effect.

The first major applications of Buddhist-influenced psychotherapy were based on various forms of meditation, a term that may sound a bit religious, which is really a sort of catch-all for a variety of methods used to train our minds. These methods share a common theme, which involves the training of a greater, non-judgemental, accepting experience of our inner life. Meditation is simply a way of slowing down and paying attention to what's going on in our minds, right now. Sometimes we might meditate by drawing our attention to specific things such as our breathing, a flower or a candle, or the act of walking. In Western applications, these types of meditations are often guided by a teacher or a recording. As we begin to take a look at these ideas of meditation, I invite you to consider that willingness and practice will help open your awareness, help you get in touch with the present moment and that no spiritual beliefs, mystical assumptions, or magical thinking are involved.

One of the pioneers of this work is the Massachusetts Institute of Technology (MIT)-trained molecular biologist, Jon Kabat-Zinn, who is also a student of the Zen master, Seung Sahn. Over the past twenty years, Jon has made a major contribution to Western healthcare by combining his knowledge of Buddhism with his knowledge of Western biology, and by developing ways to teach meditation and other skills in Western medical contexts. Originally, Kabat-Zinn was interested in how he could help people with chronic pain and terminal illness, for whom conventional medicine had little further to offer. He found that if people learned to shift into a focused, flexible and non-judgemental mode of awareness, and were able to remain in the presence of their discomfort or fear with a gentle and open-hearted acceptance, their pain often became more bearable, and their lives more liveable. Kabat-Zinn went on to help develop a 'Mindfulness-Based Stress Reduction' (MBSR) programme for people suffering from chronic physical illness and pain conditions.[5]

Researched-based evidence now supports the idea that MBSR and other similar techniques can help us cope not only with physical pain but also with difficult feelings and challenging experiences, and can help patients reduce their experience of stress and anxiety. The concepts of mindfulness and acceptance are now part of a new range of therapies such as ACT,[6] DBT, Mindfulness-Based Cognitive Therapy (MBCT) and CFT. My website, www.mindfulcompassion.com, is a good place to start if you want to find out more about these therapies.

An Introduction to Mindfulness

The core of many of these newer approaches in psychotherapy is known as 'mindfulness', which is important to the development of compassion and refers to a 2,500-year-old method for training the mind to cultivate a particular way of paying attention.

Cultivating mindfulness can help make us aware of just how much our minds and our attention are floating around on a current of different feelings and desires. Our attention can bob about like a cork on choppy seas but if you sit quietly for a moment, allow your breath to find its own rhythm and pace, rest in that breath, and let your mind settle into the experience of breathing, you will notice that it quickly moves away from the focus on your breathing and turns to other things. For example, you may start to think about what you've got to do tomorrow, what to sort out for dinner, what Aunt Ethel said about your new dress, and so on. This is sometimes called 'automatic pilot' or 'monkey mind'. It is completely natural and relates to our 'always on, better-safe-than-sorry' problem-solving machine and threat-detection system, which is easily activated and which can dominate our behaviour, our attention, and seize control of our consciousness. After all, that's what it is designed to do.

Mindfulness is a way of noticing how our attention gets pulled in different directions and it is a way of practising the gentle, persistent art of returning our attention to the present moment. Mindfulness training has been demonstrated to be an effective treatment for a range of psychological problems such as depressive relapse, anxiety and emotion regulation difficulties.[7] By developing our ability to be mindful, and learning how to apply mindfulness to more healthy methods of coping with stress, we may become able to break our habitual and unhelpful responses to anxiety.[8]

If you have ever walked in a forest on a cool and cloudy night, without even the glow of the moon to guide your way, you may understand what it is to be truly in the dark. The shadows of the trees obscure whatever light there is. All around you, the limits of your vision give way to blackness that may cause you to freeze in your tracks, or nervously feel your way forward. The uncertainty of this sensory void might grab hold of your behaviour, and narrow your options for moving to very few possible courses. The limited perception may be thrilling and challenging, or it may be frightening and debilitating.

What if you could see in the dark? Not by bringing more light into the environment, but by possessing an ability to see through the darkness in a kind of infrared way that would allow you to see a richer palate of colours than could have imagined possible. You could run and hurdle your way through this environment the way you might on a bright, calm spring day. Your actions would be your own again. No more feeling around in the dark.

We have discussed in the previous chapters how our minds have evolved with the capacity to relate one experience to any other experience. This weaves a web together from everything we have ever known, allowing one thought or emotion to ceaselessly trigger another. When they unfold before us, we experience these thoughts and emotions as if they were real and true, and this allows the random associations of our imagination to seize control of our feelings and behaviours and, in fact, of our lives. We have also discussed how the more we try to push our thoughts and feelings away, the stronger they become.

However, our ability to clearly see the world around us, with all of its possibilities and meanings, is obscured by the content of our minds, very much as our vision is obscured by the dark that surrounds us in the forest. Our range of available behaviours narrows as we grope around, treading carefully. We become enveloped and enshrouded by the uncertainty of our futures, the regrets of our past, and the ceaseless struggle to rid ourselves of pain and suffering due to our anxiety.

But, again, what if we could see in the dark? Not by changing the contents of our thoughts, or by altering our internal environment, nor by dispelling the dark, the experience of pain, the universality of human suffering or the finitude of life, but by cultivating the capacity to see clearly by being open and able to feel things for what they are.

We broaden our possibilities as we become more able to see through the darkness, and rid ourselves of our attachment to our own past stories or the way we've judged ourselves. We become more able to move with more freedom through our lives, with passion, dignity and abandon, towards what matters most to us, as freely as we could move through the forest on the spring day.

From Mindfulness to Compassion: CFT

Along with mindfulness, one of the other great traditions of the East is the deliberate development of compassion for all living beings. The Dalai Lama, for example, points out that compassion can quite literally transform our minds.[9]

We discussed earlier how compassion from other people has a calming effect on us: when we are upset because of frightening or saddening circumstances we turn to our partners or friends for help, support and attention. They listen carefully, validate our feelings and make it clear that they will do what they can to help. We become secure in the knowledge that they care about what happens to us, that they are not condemning us and that they are kind. How does this make you feel? But how would you feel if you asked for help from someone you care about and they seemed quite dismissive and disinterested, not only by what they said but also by their body language? What if they gave you the distinct impression that they might even blame or judge you for having such problems in the first place?

We all have an intuitive wisdom that loving kindness, support and compassion help us to bear our suffering, and that criticism, neglect, shaming and blaming usually make things much worse. This is true of self-criticism as well!

Many years ago, my friend and colleague Paul Gilbert noticed that some of his clients became very self-critical or ashamed when they were distressed: they were good at kicking themselves when they were down. Paul found that he couldn't always help them by challenging their negative thinking, or by teaching them mindfulness; however, when he taught them to be kind to themselves he could often help them move away from their focus on self-condemnation. Some people were afraid of being kind to themselves, and feared any form of self-compassion; however, even when we have learned to be distrustful of the concept of compassion, such as when our caregivers have been abusive or neglectful, mind training can help us 'unlearn' this notion and begin to free us from anxiety and destructive emotions.

Paul was inspired to develop a form of compassionate mind training based on his observations and his understanding of inherent biological soothing processes that can create a new relationship with our anxiety, and with our shame and self-criticism. Self-compassion can allow us room to feel the pain and complexity of our emotions, which we may need to confront so that our anxiety loosens its grip. This may be painful, and complicated, but when we develop a basic orientation to be helpful, supportive, kind and accepting towards ourselves we may be able to deal with, and more importantly, tolerate, our distress better, and have more control over the direction of our behaviour and our lives. The Compassion Focused Therapy approach to anxiety is based upon this basic idea.

Compassion is more than just kindness, and involves a range of attributes, qualities and capacities. The Dalai Lama defines it as a sensitivity to the suffering of others with a commitment to do something about it. He points to two key elements: attention (sensitivity) and motivation (commitment). The approach to compassion we will develop here incorporates these insights. We should also note that over 2,600 years ago the teacher known as 'The Buddha' (which is Sanskrit for 'The One Who Woke Up') talked in terms of an eight-fold pathway for the cultivation of compassion involving attention, thinking, speech, livelihood and action. Developing scientific-based approaches to the cultivation of compassion is fundamental to what we call Compassion Focused Therapy (CFT) and compassionate mind training. CFT involves the therapeutic relationship and a way of thinking about psychological problems; compassionate mind training refers to specific exercises that anybody can use to train their minds to develop compassionate qualities.

CFT is linked to Buddhist approaches to mindfulness; for example, in the Mahayana tradition, compassion is seen as having a central transformational power and trains people in particular kinds of attention, thinking, feeling and behaviour to help them transform their experiences of things such as anxiety. CFT shares part of this approach, in that specific methods are used to bring about changes in attention, emotions and compassionate action. However, unlike traditional Buddhism, CFT is also based on evolutionary psychology and neuroscience.

When Paul Gilbert was developing his therapy techniques, he noticed that shame and self-criticism were often triggered by experiences of anxiety and distress, and interfered with his patients' ability to move towards their goals in therapy. As a result, one of the central aims of CFT is to help people address the shame and blame they may heap upon themselves in response to anxiety and distress. CFT emphasizes that we have emerged from an evolutionary process, as a part of the flow of life on our planet. We did not choose to be here; we did not choose our families, the cultures we were born into, or the many elements of our history that have shaped who we are. In a very real sense, who we have become and what we are experiencing is not our design and, again, not our fault; however it's important not to collapse into a heap of 'giving up' but to see this as the beginning of moving towards a fuller understanding of ourselves and taking responsibility for our lives. We have the ability to think about and make decisions about how we want our minds to be developed – in the same way we make decisions about how we develop and train our bodies. If we do nothing and simply lie around and eat anything available, whenever we fancy it, we will become fat and unhealthy. But knowing this gives us the option to learn about our diet and the importance of exercise. It is the same with our minds: knowing how tricky they are and sensitive to anxiety gives us the option to learn how to cope with anxiety. We may choose to take responsibility for the course of our lives but also we must bear in mind that suffering is a universal part of the human condition, that anxiety is a natural and unavoidable part of the human experience. If we are worried, or agitated, panicked or desperate, we can take some comfort in remembering that this is not our fault. By doing so, we can see anxiety as a natural part of our design and then learn that we can respond to our anxiety by taking a mindful and accepting mental stance. We can respond by doing things that will help us cope, rather than by habitually responding in ways that can actually make things worse such as trying to suppress our experiences, misusing drugs and alcohol, or adopting a self-critical attitude.

Creating Inner Compassion and the Attachment System

The CFT model is based on research showing that some of the ways in which we instinctively regulate our response to threats have evolved from the attachment system that operates between infant and mother, and other basic relationships between mutually supportive people. We have specific systems in our brain that are sensitive to the kindness of others, and the experience of this kindness has a major impact on the way we process these threats, and the way we process anxiety in particular.

Two of the most significant twentieth-century psychologists, John Bowlby and Mary Ainsworth, observed that the attachment bond between a caregiver and an infant provides more than just protection, feeding and learning opportunities. It also provides what is known as a 'secure base', which functions as a place that is soothing and calming in the presence of distressing emotions or potential environment threats. This secure base is one aspect of our behaviour that's been passed down to us as we've evolved and it has served us well. It is natural for us to turn to emotionally significant people in our lives, and even to our internal representations of them, when we feel threatened, agitated or overwhelmed. In the 1980s Paul Gilbert was interested in the internal mechanisms that help us feel safe and the way these feelings of safety interact with those associated with threat. He understood that if children and adults were able to be calmed by the presence of supportive or caring others, there had to be a direct link between support and the experience of threat. So, after much research, he labelled our physiological systems that switch on these feelings of safety as the 'social-safeness system'. These include our responsiveness to certain communicative behaviours such as facial expressions, tone of voice, touch, and the accessibility or proximity of our significant attachment figures. The activation of attuned, secure, soothing relationships affords us this secure base, which then allows us to interact with our environment with greater confidence when we face challenges, and return to a sense of safety and protection in this secure base when necessary. There is a connection between feeling safe and being able to explore. This is important because, as we will see, there is a close interaction between mindfulness, which allows you to have open and explorative attention, and a feeling of safety.

The process of establishing a secure base and attachments involves a special set of brain cells known as 'mirror neurons', which allow us to observe the emotions of others, and literally feel what they are feeling. According to Daniel Goleman, mirror neurons 'act as a neural WiFi, attuning to the other person's internal state moment to moment and recreating that state in our own brain – their emotions, their movements, their intentions. This means [that a feeling such as] empathy is based not just on reading the external signs of someone else's feeling, like the hint of a frown, or the irritation in their voice. Because of mirror neurons, we feel with the other. Empathy, then, includes attuning to our own feelings in order to better sense what's going on with the other person.'[10]

According to attachment theory, secure relationships with others allow us to better cope with and manage the range of difficult emotions that arise in response to inner and outer circumstances. When we are threatened, our attachment system is activated and we seek to be close to and gain comfort from a significant person in our lives. This sort of relationship is referred to as an 'attachment relationship'. The person who is the object of attachment is sometimes referred to as an 'attachment figure', who may help us cope with the perceived threats in our environment, and access our positive emotions.

Of course there are differences from person to person in how effectively, or consistently, this attachment system functions. Those of us who are raised with stable, secure attachment relationships may be more likely to be resilient, flexible and have an increased capacity to cope with difficult emotions.[11] Those of us who experience neglect, trauma, abuse, or even just a generally inconsistent and emotionally unavailable attachment relationship to our caregiver, may be more likely to have difficulty with coping, with the ability to be reflective and thoughtful, and have a hard time soothing ourselves. A person who can activate, even if symbolically, their attachment and affiliation system to respond to difficult emotions may have an easier time with self-compassion. Studies suggest that a person who has a secure attachment system may put more focus of their attention and resources upon generating positive emotions, upon problem-solving or shifting their perspective on events than would a person with an unreliable, anxious or avoidance style of attachment.[12]

Additionally, and on the biological side, we have certain hormones such as oxytocin that are linked to affiliation[13] and which help us downgrade threat processing, in the ways kindness and self-compassion can soothe us when we are fearful. When we practise self-compassion for long periods of time, it seems that regions of the brain that involve self-soothing and positive emotions are activated more easily, particularly in the face of stress;[14] thus, they help us cope with anxiety.

The key idea in CFT is to specifically train our minds to focus on compassion, and to activate compassionate ways of responding to our anxiety to better regulate our feelings. By doing so, we are stimulating specific biological systems in our brain designed to calm down the threat system. I can show you this with a simple diagram that we use in CFT.

If your mind is focused on worrying or thinking too much about certain things, over and over again, on being self-critical or on various other anxious themes, it will simply stimulate your threat system and cause you to get locked in to stimulating your threat system. It's possible though to step out of that by redirecting your thoughts, attention or by becoming mindful. The idea is to break the link between what your new brain is doing and how it is stimulating old-brain threat systems. Part of the essence of CFT is using parts of our minds, including the affiliation system, which have evolved with the specific purpose of calming down the threat system. After all, there are direct connections between these two.

Basic evolved system in our brain

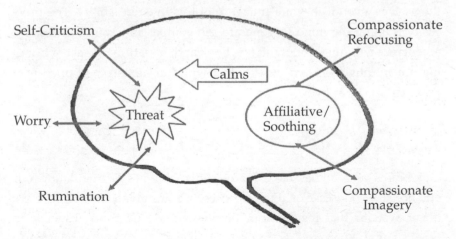

From *Compassion Focused Therapy: Distinctive Features*, Gilbert, 2010; reprinted with permission of Routledge.

While modern living largely has enabled us to free ourselves from threats such as the fear of predators, certain childhood diseases, and to some extent food shortages, it does, however, provide an array of other types of threats. We live in a world now surrounded by a strangers, whereas most primates including early humans operated in small groups of others who were familiar to us. We now also live in a world of constant social comparison and in fear of being seen as inferior. Early human childcare was based on multiple caregivers, involving extended family members such as grandmothers, siblings and friends. This is less true today when many families are smaller or living apart. For many areas of our lives, there is something of a mismatch between the environment that affected our evolution and the environment that we are surrounded by now; this increases our vulnerability to a whole range of anxieties. Our understanding of the reasons for this discord and subsequent increase in anxiety can facilitate social change. It can also help us understand that our vulnerability to anxiety is not our fault.

The location of my practice in the heart of New York City means that, in the middle of relative abundance and safety, I regularly meet people whose minds have conjured innumerable terrors. Thankfully, each of these clients possess the wisdom of self-compassion and ability to soothe themselves, even if they are unaware of this inherent ability. The process of training the mind to generate self-compassion, mindfulness and acceptance will run throughout this book and, hopefully, the act of bringing our intuitive wisdom into contact with our anxiety will open new possibilities in our lives.

The Three-Circle Model of Emotion Regulation

Our brains and bodies have many different ways of regulating our emotional responses. For our purposes, we are going to look at three major systems that regulate our emotions and affect our response to what's going on around us. In CFT, these systems are often referred to as the 'three-circle model', as we like to represent them as three circles of different colours, which is a representation of the most important areas involved in human emotional response. The illustration below shows these three circles and how they interact:

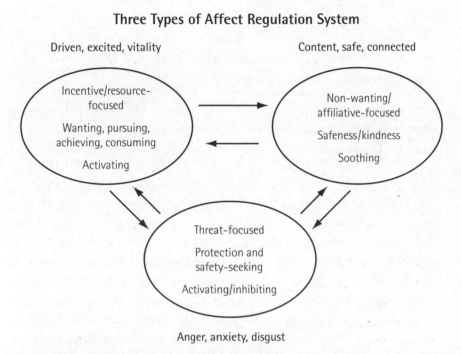

Three Types of Affect Regulation System

From Gilbert, 2009, *The Compassionate Mind*; reprinted with permission.

In the past thirty years or so our understanding of how the brain creates and regulates emotion has advanced enormously. It's long been known that we have a system in our brains that enables us to detect and respond to threats.[15] What's become more evident recently is that we also have different types of positive emotion: one kind is associated with drive and achievement, doing and acquiring; another is associated with inner calmness, and a sense of peaceful well-being. When we're not stimulating the drive and threat systems – as everyday life does all the time – the mind settles and this second type of emotion can come through; these are linked to endorphins and hormones such as oxytocin, which may have evolved with the attachment system.

This is a simplified example of the use of neuroscience but it's helpful to think about what we're trying to do with our brains when we practise compassion. Keep in mind that these systems are constantly interacting. It may be a good idea to think of them as if they were colours that were constantly mixing to create new colours which, when applied to a canvas, can create different shapes, patterns and balances. Let's look at these systems, or circles, in more detail.

Threat-Detection and Safety-Seeking System

We have seen the ways this system can act upon us to influence our attention, thinking, emotions and behaviours and how we have evolved with the capacity to detect threats quickly. Our threat-detection system doesn't need to be activated by a direct threat to our well-being – if our loved ones or companions also face danger, this threat-detection system may kick in to action. It also may be activated by social threats, such as separation from the group, which can make us feel vulnerable to attack. Similarly, it may be activated if we feel threatened by the risk of rejection or abandonment by others in our family or social group.

The threat-detection system involves the processing of sensory information to sight, sound, smell, taste and touch, and sends signals to our brain, which then stimulates certain areas in our emotional processing regions, the limbic system, if we sense danger.[16] In particular, the amygdala, a cluster of nerve cells located on either side of the brain, becomes activated very rapidly, sending information to another part of our brain, the hypothalamus, which activates our stress response. The hypothalamus then communicates with the adrenal gland, and our body becomes ready for danger and starts to produce adrenaline and cortisol, a hormone released in response to stress. In an instant, when faced with a potential threat, real or imagined, we are ready for action.

Generally, this is not a favourite circle for people to hang out in for prolonged periods of time; however, if you have struggled with an anxiety disorder, this may feel all too familiar to you.

Drive and Resource-Acquisition System

For a moment, imagine that an email popped up on your computer or phone as you were reading this book. The email was from your spouse or partner, who informs you that, although you hadn't been aware of it, the two of you had bought a lottery ticket and, amazingly, you have won the largest prize in history. Within a week hundreds of millions of pounds will be transferred into your bank account. This isn't some Internet scam involving oil inheritance from West Africa, but a real stroke of brilliant luck, which has now made you instantly, fabulously wealthy. You imagine how you might use this untold wealth, the places you would visit, the things that you would buy – items of luxury and items of necessity. You now immediately have all the power that unfathomable wealth can bring. Can you imagine what that excitement would feel like coursing through your body, as you realized that all of your financial troubles have immediately evaporated? If you can, that rush and thrill represents the activation of something called the 'incentive-focused emotion-regulation system'. Our positive emotions, such as those that correspond to a sense of thrill or ecstasy, are involved in our seeking out those things that will help us survive or enhance our experience.[17] All the things we do for pleasure, such as seeking the perfect meal, the best vacation or exciting sexual experiences, and our drive to win, to celebrate, and to revel in being alive, are all expressions of this system.

Although much of this may seem positive, it can also turn fairly negative if the incentive- focus system becomes too dominant. For example, people who experience manic episodes can have their lives dominated by excessively expansive or related moods. Their sense of themselves can swell, and they can find themselves obsessively seeking out intense pleasure despite high risks. They may not be able to sleep, or they may become completely engulfed by goal-orientated pursuits. People with addictions may also face an overly active incentive-focus system. Our thoughts can race under such conditions, our impulses difficult to restrain, and our lives unmanageable.

This system involves a neurochemical called dopamine,[18] which is related to our experience of being driven to do things. Many different human experiences involve an increase in dopamine, such as the intense experience of falling in love, or going to an all-night rave, or cheering as your team advances towards winning the World Cup. Activation of dopamine is absolutely essential for human survival, but an overabundance can lead to problems.

The way we function does not involve one emotion-regulation system ruling the roost over the others, and to function as a flexible, healthy and adaptive person our aim should be to achieve a better balance among these different emotion-regulation systems.

Social Safety and Soothing Systems

When babies are born, they are unable to defend themselves and are absolutely dependent upon their caregivers for survival. When I was a boy, I remember watching a film of the birth of a foal. Very shortly after it was born it was up and running, as if it were born knowing most of what it needed to know, and had the capacity to quickly engage with its environment. But when we think of children in the first few weeks of their lives, perhaps even well into their twenties, we can begin to understand how much help, protection, support and guidance they need to help them develop their soothing and contentment system so that they can go out to explore the world.

The hormone oxytocin is also involved in a feeling of happiness that arises when we feel safe, connected and loved by others. The activation of compassion within ourselves is very much related to this soothing and contentment system.[19] If our threat-detection system evolved as a way for us to protect ourselves, then the soothing and contentment system has also evolved as a way for us to protect ourselves through caring, kind and supportive attachment bonds.[20] Our compassion for ourselves and others appears to emerge through the evolution of our affiliations and our ability to regulate our emotions draws upon our sense of safety, contentment and an awareness of our connection to others.

We are just beginning to understand the soothing contentment system. What is our sense of contentment made of? Older psychological models of happiness, such as those derived from dear old Sigmund Freud, often looked at the reduction of our subconscious driving forces. Other models looked at the ways our threat-detection systems could be tweaked, or simple reward schedules met to help us become satisfied; however, current research points us in another direction. It appears that we have a specific emotional system that allows us to experience peacefulness, contentment and well-being. Certain states of mind allow the body to release neurochemicals that directly involve a sense of soothing. When we find ourselves in situations that activate these chemicals, such as when we're in the calming presence of a nurturing, wise and beloved family member, our soothing and contentment system is directly utilizing neurochemistry that supports and enables these feelings. Far from a mere blissed-out warmth, the activation of the soothing and contentment system can involve a subjective sense of peacefulness, clarity of mind and insight. This is not due to just an absence of anxiety and fear; it is also due to strong, moving and potential transformational experiences of positive emotions.

Compassionate mind training aims to help us focus on and then easily access our experiences of contentment, self-soothing, and safety. We can use many methods, ranging from visualization and meditation to changes in behaviour that lead to greater self-care and cultivate our capacity for compassion. All of these methods involve the deliberate activation of the soothing and contentment system, which has evolved from the way mammals care for their young, and from the emotional bond between parent and child.

As you probably know, the principle that underlies our understanding of evolution is known as natural selection, whereby the traits and behaviours that promote the survival and flourishing of a species tend to be passed from generation to generation, and those traits that don't lead to survival will die off. From this point of view, what are the evolutionary functions of the human behaviour that we would describe as 'caring for one another'? Well, most obviously, caring for our young allows them the greatest chances of survival, and to then pass their own genetic code to subsequent generations. Beyond this, bonds among families, friends and kinspeople have allowed human beings to form groups, cooperate, and protect the survival and well-being of the group. Emerging from these behaviours are friendship, empathy and altruism.

Among mammals, the emotional systems related to soothing and content-ment begin to take on new functions that weren't present in evolutionary history. For warm-blooded mammals this system, which communicates an experience of safety, begins to involve a dual function of the experi-ence of affection, affiliation and care, the production of a sense of calm and a decrease of our threat-detection system.

When we view the evolution of caregiving and its relationship to the soothing and contentment system we can begin to make sense of the fact that while mammals have fewer offspring than many other species it is far more important that these offspring survive to avoid extinction. You might see evolution as life playing out myriad options, exploring and evolving different ways to flourish and grow, in ever more complex and efficient ways. When Paul Gilbert describes evolution as a flow of life he is being far more than poetic. There is a literal, physical transformation of the raw stuff of life on earth, of the minerals, energy and proteins derived from far-flung stardust into our proteins, amino acids and DNA, then into the variety of species that give birth to one another, survive, and change over hundreds of millions of years.

Mammalian parents care for and invest in their young, providing the 'secure base' we mentioned earlier, which allows offspring to safely examine their environment and then return to a protected, secure base. And with the arrival of early primates, and eventually human, caregiver behaviours, we can begin to see the emergence of the soothing function of the attachment bond between the caregiver and child that serves as the foundation for the 'compassionate mind': human caregiving emerges as a complex blend of emotions, motivations and behavioural tendencies that result in social mentalities with effects that are unique to humans.

Contemporary and Ancient Concepts of Compassion

Compassion is an ancient concept. We find it in the earliest of human writings, such as the RigVeda, a beautiful epic poem that is perhaps over 10,000 years old and which was created by the earliest civilized people of Central Asia. When great civilizations transformed from eras of subjugation and oppression to epochs of abundance and prosperity, the shift involved a movement towards compassion and interpersonal empathy.[21] The roots of the world's great religions and wisdom traditions such as Christianity, Judaism, Islam, Hinduism, and particularly Buddhism, have emphasized compassion as a source of the alleviation of suffering. Western science, the dominant way of thinking in our present era, has now come to recognize compassion as one of the central processes in the alleviation of human suffering and its involvement in our emotional well-being. It is an emerging evolutionary process, with a purpose and an essentially human character and has a measurable effect on the human mind and body.

All of us want pleasant feelings, and to rid ourselves of feelings of pain, displeasure and anxiety. That just makes perfect sense. But what is the value of soothing above and beyond just feeling good? What purpose might this ability to regulate our emotions through mindful compassion serve? Courage, that is one of its key purposes – to give us courage, without which we would not be able to put into action what is needed to calm and soothe ourselves, to confront our demons both inside us and outside. The loving parent keeps their child out of danger but also encourages the child to face up to the challenges of the world by learning how to experience anxiety and deal with it. So, compassion is intimately linked to courage and the ability to face up to the things we fear. And you can find that courage within yourself more easily if you create a calm, understanding and encouraging voice in your head. That is the simple message: train your mind to be compassionate and you will allow yourself the space to be able to do those things you need to do in order to deal with your anxiety.

I'd like to ask you now to use your imagination to notice how compassion and mindfulness might serve a broader purpose. Let's imagine that you are the captain of an old-fashioned wooden sailing ship. The masts creak and only the wind behind your sails keeps you moving. There are no computers, there is no GPS, and you have only yourself, your keen eye and your sense of direction to guide you. Imagine that you are sailing this ship towards whatever it is that you value most in your life: ahead, just on the horizon – you can see it – that aim that will allow you to feel fulfilled, purposeful and vital. Whatever that is for you, right here and now, is waiting on that horizon. You have sailed this ship for a very long time, and you are confident she is seaworthy. Over the years, you have seen just how much stress and strain she can withstand. Nevertheless, tonight the sea is churning. All around you dark clouds and white-capped waves are swirling and a storm threatens. This storm is your anxiety. Jolts of electricity crackle off of the water, just as your nervous system revs up in the presence of imaginary threats. The crew shouts warnings and fearful cries to you, just as you can envision for yourself various horrible possible consequences of shipwreck. You are surrounded by the storm of your anxiety. How can you remain calm enough to sail this ship home to what matters most to you? If you turn back, you turn away from a life well lived. If you stop, the storm threatens to engulf you. You choose to carry on. Right here and right now, you can choose to bring your full, flexible and focused attention to the present moment, through the practice of mindful awareness. Just as you, the captain, love your ship and crew, and put their well-being before yourself and can steel your determination, so too can you access a great wellspring of care and acceptance for yourself, through training your compassionate mind. In time, you can learn to activate your intuitive wisdom, access your mindful compassion, and remain calm in the storm of anxiety, as you move forward in the direction of your own valued aims.

This ability to remain calm in the storm is not only available to you, but is designed to be an essential part of what it means to be human. Many people have been aware of this for a long time and, fortunately, they have recorded a log of their own voyages and left a course for us to follow.

As we approach a deeper understanding of the role of compassion in emotion regulation, let's take a look at what Western psychologists and scientists have to say about the situation. Compassion's essence can be found in basic human kindness, with a deep awareness of the suffering of oneself and of other living beings, coupled with a wish and an effort to relieve this suffering. This definition lays the groundwork for CFT and research has found that training people in developing a compassionate mind in a gradual, structured way can reduce depression, help lessen shame and self-criticism, and can help patients deal with difficult emotions such as anxiety.

Compassion is not just an emotion; it is also a multi-purpose system and strategy for functioning and interacting with the world. Many aspects of being human, such as thinking, the experience of emotions, overt behaviours, and the deployment of attention are all coordinated and activated by compassion in what CFT refers to as a social mentality,[22] which is a blend of thoughts, emotions, and actions that guide our motivation. Social mentalities also direct and affect our attention, thoughts, and behaviours as we seek out and maintain relationships with others and are involved in the positive feelings that arise when our relationships are working for us. They are also involved, however, in our experience of negative emotions that show up when our relationships aren't working.

Archetypes and Self-Compassion

The idea of an archetype has its origins in the writings of the psychiatrist Carl Jung, who noted that archetypes represent innate frameworks and prototypes for understanding ourselves and our environment. These prototypes might not exist in the forefront of our awareness, but they influence us nevertheless via our unconscious to inform our thoughts, feelings and behaviours. Examples might be found in the prototype of 'the mother' or 'the hero'. Across cultures, languages, social structures and historical periods such prototypes emerge in myth, social roles, and in the stories we make up in our own minds about the world. Archetypes represent 'the source of the repeating desires and relationships that echo down through history'.[23] But social mentality, which we touched on earlier, demystifies the concept of the archetype by viewing such patterns as naturally selected strategies that have evolved to guide our feelings, thoughts and behaviours towards the best way to adapt and interact with our environment. So, when we are training ourselves to cultivate our minds to be compassionate, we are actually activating and then developing an innate social mentality.

Another leading Western researcher on compassion, Kristen Neff, has emphasized a theory of 'self-compassion'[24] which is different from either self-esteem or compassion for others. Self-compassion involves three primary elements: self-kindness, an awareness of our common humanity and mindful awareness. It has been shown that higher levels of self-compassion have been found to correlate with lower levels of depression and anxiety. Such research has also demonstrated positive correlations between self-compassion and a range of other desirable experiences, such as enhanced life satisfaction, feelings of social connectedness, a sense of personal initiative and other positive emotions.[25]

It has been suggested that we have evolved to be able to preserve both ourselves and our genetic relatives and that we may have different emotional systems that guide our own survival and the survival of humanity as a group. The species-preservation emotion system is thought to have evolved from the loving bond between the nurturing mother and the dependent children, who were more likely to survive under the care and attention of loving and dedicated parents than under the care of neglectful or inadequate parents. Over millions of years, those qualities of nurturing, kindness and care gradually emerged as central and essential aspects of our survival. As a result, we have evolved to feel soothed and feel safe in the presence of kindness, care and loving attention. In turn, our sense of compassion has evolved into one of the major systems we use to regulate our emotions.

Buddhist Models of Compassion

While Western thinkers adopted an outward-looking perspective, crafting technologies and scientific methods that would influence our physical, outer dimensions of interaction with the environment, Eastern thinkers devoted generations of effort to mapping and understanding the inner-looking perspective of mental and emotional experience. If you are reading this, and you are thinking that I sound like a Buddhist preacher, or a new-age philosopher, I don't blame you at all. The very idea that reliable, scientific solutions to psychological problems might emerge from spiritual tradition would have sounded ludicrous to many other people just a few years ago. However, scientific data continues to prove that Buddhist psychology has produced effective ways for us to alleviate human suffering, not only by altering our behaviour and emotions, but also by actually changing the function and structure of the human brain itself.[26] So, when we turn to Buddhist psychology as a starting point in our understanding of the nature of compassion, we turn to it with a confident knowledge that thousands of years of scholarship and meditative practice have provided us with a legacy of unparalleled wisdom about the nature of our minds and our emotions.

Buddhist psychology expounds the idea that we all live our lives through the veil of our own imagination, thoughts, feelings and emotional memories and that as much as we might strive to see things as they 'really are' our inner world filters and distorts our perception. The aim of Buddhist psychology is to train the mind to experience reality as directly and clearly as is possible, moment by moment. In doing so, and in coming to accept reality just as it is, we can take a broader view of reality, and become less attached to and stuck within our pain and suffering.

Generations of Buddhists have asserted that four aspects of compassion might be the central ingredients of our individual spiritual evolution.[27] Let's take a look at these four in some depth.

The first aspect is described by the ancient Sanskrit term *'Metta'*, which refers to a feeling of loving kindness for ourselves and for others and which represents a warm, friendly and loving feeling and means that we aspire for happiness, both for ourselves and for others. This particular concept is crucial to an important and widely practised meditation based upon cultivating just this quality of Metta. Later we will look at this technique in some depth, and you will learn exactly how you can cultivate this quality for yourself.

Buddhist meditators have long believed that a gradual development of Metta is essential to our well-being and personal evolution. Recently, there have been some exciting studies that seem to support this view and which have used neuro-imaging to examine the brain functions and structures of long-term practitioners of compassion meditation.[28] It has been shown that advanced, compassion-focused meditators respond to distressing images and events with an increased activation of brain regions involved in empathy, love and positive emotions. This supports Paul Gilbert's assertion that compassionate mind training can result in a shift in our method of emotion regulation from reliance upon the threat-focused response system to the affiliative, compassion-oriented soothing system. It appears that regular practice in developing loving kindness may actually relate to changes in the brain that can help us deal better with stress and difficult emotions.

The second form of compassion that is discussed by Buddhist psychology is referred to as *'Karuna'*, which is typically translated directly as 'compassion' and which involves a heartfelt aspiration for all beings to be free from suffering. Beyond this aspiration or motivation, Karuna relates to the clarification of compassion as a value that guides and informs our behaviour. Those who are cultivating Karuna are engaged in an ongoing commitment to ethical behaviour that serves the value of compassion, and leads to happiness being shared and nurtured. As a result, those who are practising Karuna engage in a process related to actively bearing the suffering of others; indeed, modern behavioural research has found that by simply acknowledging that we can feel each other's pain is crucial to our ability to be more sympathetic and understanding. An element of Karuna will be involved in our work to train our minds to be more compassionate.

The third form of Buddhist compassion is known as 'Mudita', which describes a sense of joy that arrives when we appreciate the well-being and happiness of others and it is believed to be an inexhaustible source of inner happiness that can be accessed through mental training. In some Buddhist teaching sources, Mudita is related to the feeling of deep happiness that parents take in the flourishing of their children. Jealousy, envy, and the addictive pursuit of pleasure are considered to be the opposites of Mudita, and activation of these emotions is seen as a block to the experience of Mudita. The goals of developing Mudita relate to the goals of CFT, which aims to teach us how to deliberately come into contact with a sense of compassion in order to regulate other, destructive emotions.

The fourth from of compassion that is discussed in the earliest texts of classical Buddhist psychology is known as 'Upekkha', most directly translated as 'equanimity', an ability to meet both the good and the bad in life with an attitude of acceptance, willingness, calmness and understanding. Just such an attitude of mindful acceptance and a willingness to embrace the whole of life, from the rough to the smooth, has emerged in the most advanced research in psychotherapy as an essential element in the process of emotional healing. As we begin to learn about training our compassionate mind, we will see how cultivating acceptance of things just as they are enables us to experience joy and freedom more readily.

These four elements are the building blocks of human happiness; however, there is one more aspect of the Buddhist concept of compassion that I'd like to discuss: the 'Bodhicitta'.[29]

Bodhicitta is usually referred to as a passionate and selfless desire for the end of suffering of all beings; however, I like to remember what the roots of the word mean. 'Bodhi' means 'waking up' and 'Citta' means 'mind'. Many practitioners of Mahayana Buddhism believe that regular practice of gentle yet disciplined mental training will result in the possibility that all beings can be free from suffering, and that this possibility is a natural part of our waking up to the reality of the human condition. Bodhicitta relates to the wisdom of knowing how interconnected we are to one another.

5 The First Turning of the Wheel of Compassion: Exploring the Attributes and Skills of the Compassionate Mind

Contrasting the Anxious Mind and the Compassionate Mind

In our earlier discussion we learned how anxiety affects such things as our attention, thinking, behaviour, emotions, our imagination and motivation. We also learned that our affiliation and compassion system can be activated to stimulate our compassionate mind and change our mental state so that we have a calmer and more soothing way to deal with our experiences, good or bad.

The diagrams below illustrate how two different types of brain patterns – the 'threatened mind' and the 'compassionate mind' – can affect the way we feel. Let's look at how the activation of your 'threatened mind' might result in a different experience than the activation of your 'compassionate mind'. Imagine that you've had a history of feeling anxious in social situations, and that it is your first day at university. Your whole day will be scheduled with events during freshers' week, where you will be meeting new people, and be expected to form new relationships, ask questions, start conversations, and basically be faced with a host of different social challenges. This is the sort of thing you've dreaded over the course of your entire life, but it is something you have to face today. Even before this day begins, perhaps while tossing and turning in bed the previous night, your threat-detection system will be active and will be creating a state of anxiety, worry and fear.

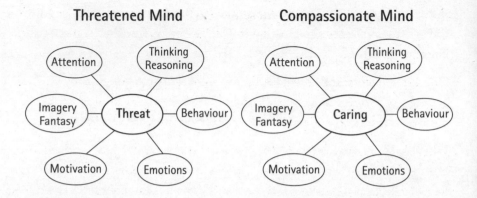

From Gilbert, 2010, *Overcoming Depression*; reprinted with permission.

The threat-detection system will affect what we *attend* to in our environment; for example, we might scan the faces of the people at the orientation to see if there is any evidence of disapproval. Our threatened minds might focus on hypothetical situations where we embarrass ourselves or say the wrong thing. Our attention might become fixed on past social experiences that have led to feelings of humiliation or rejection. The activation of our threat-detection system narrows our attention, narrows what we attend to, and keeps us feeling anxious.

When our compassionate mind is activated, we deploy our attention differently. Yes, we might be focused partly on some feelings of anxiety; however, our compassion allows us to mindfully make space for this and remember that these feelings are a natural part of the human condition, and not our fault. The compassionate mind allows us to be kind to ourselves, and truly wish the best for ourselves, which will then allow us to feel an inner sense of safety and give us an ability to face uncertainty. Instead of focusing on the negative 'what ifs?' – 'What if that person doesn't like me?' or 'What if I spill tea down my shirt and make a fool of myself?' – our attention may turn itself instead to the likely possibility that the experience of meeting new people may be rewarding and informative. Instead of putting pressure on ourselves to perform, excel and impress, we could allow ourselves to be good enough, just as we are, in this very moment. This warm self-regard and acceptance might allow the orientation session to be what it is: a learning opportunity and a new beginning.

Our threatened mind affects how we think and reason, and generates a range of worries and predictions about how badly things could go because it is working in better-safe-than-sorry mode.

Likewise, our compassionate mind also affects how we think and reason but in a different way – one that is open more to opportunities than to fear of rejection. The compassionate mind provides a counterbalance to our threatened mind, and remembers that we aren't obliged to buy into the anxious thoughts that pop into our heads.

If we let our threatened mind dominate we may engage in certain behaviour that is based upon threat perception and a desire to find safety. So, in our example, we may feel a desire to avoid the first day of university altogether, and make up an excuse to stay at home. We may feel an urge to activate safety-seeking behaviour such as standing apart from the groups at orientation, pretending to look at our phone, avoiding eye contact, or even drinking one too many pints at lunch to 'take the edge off'. Our urge to avoid, escape, and push away our feelings of anxiety is a natural result of our threat-detection system being stimulated, and it can be very hard to withstand the pull of such urges when we are stuck in our threatened-mind mode.

In contrast, when we activate our compassionate mind in such a situation, new behavioural possibilities may present themselves. Remember: compassion gives us courage. As we try to shift from our threatened mind to our compassionate mind, we may be able to find the strength and wisdom to face our fear with mindfulness and acceptance, and more deeply engage in social interactions and new experiences. Rather than looking for ways to escape, we may focus on how to begin conversations, ask questions, and forge new relationships.

The emotions evoked by our compassionate mind are different to the emotions evoked by the threatened mind. Warmth and support are different to fear and frustration. This can feel as if a dear friend and mentor is with us, guiding us towards opportunities to live in meaningful ways and, although we are entering new and unfamiliar situations, with the help of our friend we can feel confident and secure that we can meet the challenge, and handle our happy and sad emotions with equal measure.

The threat-detection system and our threatened-mind mode can also influence our motives, which would be different if faced with a consequence of danger than with the reward of happiness and contentment. We may feel conflicted if on the one hand we value the potential good things that may result from university life but on the other hand avoid becoming involved in university life because of our anxiety.

Our compassionate mind motivates us to be kind to ourselves, to be aware of our common humanity and to allow ourselves to enjoy the present, moment by moment. Our compassionate minds are, above all, motivated to help us cope with and maybe over time even alleviate our suffering. The *motive* of the compassionate mind when we are at the university orientation day is to gently and kindly support us as we face new challenges and take new risks, so that we might live a more fulfilled and meaningful life. Our secure base, our affiliation, is within us and when we find this place of safety we can then courageously move towards our aims on that distant horizon.

The Attributes and Skills of the Compassionate Mind

Compassionate mind training employs the use of the different aspects of who we are. For example, we can build our ability to mindfully observe our thoughts and emotions with acceptance, without condemning ourselves for the way we feel, and with a sense of perspective on why we feel as we do. We can then choose to take care of ourselves, as best we can, through compassionate behaviour. Compassionate mind training involves the development of attributes and skills that, combined, help us prepare to meet the challenges of anxiety. Compassion serves as a means of bringing our emotional systems into balance and increases our sense of well-being.

In CFT we use the concept of the compassionate mind because compassion is a mind-organizing process that brings together our motives, emotions, ways of thinking, and ways of paying attention.

The circular diagram below illustrates the different aspects of the compassionate mind. In the inner ring are the core attributes of compassion and in the outer ring are the skills we can practise to develop our capacity for compassion.

Different Aspects of Compassionte Mind Training

From Gilbert, *The Compassionate Mind*, 2009; reprinted with permission.

We are going to start our journey around the circle by exploring the attribute described in this diagram as 'Care for well-being', which represents a compassionate motivation to care for ourselves and others and, as a result, to be motivated to address our problems with anxiety.

First, we must acknowledge that our struggle with anxiety is excessively distressing and may be holding us back from a life that is more content or calmer. Second, we must acknowledge that our lives can be better if we come to terms with anxiety. After all, what would be the point of learning to manage your anxiety if it would not improve the quality of your life?

To get in touch with your motivation, you might begin by writing down the benefits of working on your anxiety. If you wish, stop now, and make a list of what you would like to do if your anxiety were not the focus of your attention. What have you given up due to the struggle with anxiety? Start with small things, and move on to bigger things. This list will help you to keep your aims in life – those important things on the horizon – in the forefront of your mind and may help you remember what motivates you.

Jennifer, who we met earlier in this book, made her own list:

- If I were less focused on anxiety, I could pay more attention to developing new relationships and making new friends.

- If anxiety were less of a problem for me, I could explore new job opportunities rather than be stuck in one place.

- If I were more willing to allow myself to experience anxiety without also worrying about it so much, and to hold myself in higher regard and be kinder to myself, perhaps I could ride out the waves of panic that show up when I have a panic-stricken anxiety attack. They usually only last a couple of minutes, and they don't cause me harm, but I can lose hours and sometimes days by anticipating and then worrying about whether or not I'll have one.

Consider the kinds of things that might get in your way – maybe you have thoughts of the anxiety being too much. Or that it may be too difficult. Your brain will be acting on both fronts – to motivate you to face your anxiety and to motivate you not to. The compassionate mind approach suggests that you take a kind, understanding view of this conflict within you and then, as best as you are able, begin to think about small steps first.

Motivation waxes and wanes but it does not come out of the blue. To keep ourselves motivated, it is useful to reflect upon what we are willing to work for, suffer discomfort for, climb mountains for. You see, all of us have our mountains to climb and anxiety might be yours. Tuning in to your goals and the things that are worth working for can help you stay motivated to engage with your pain, fears and anxiety – and then you will know that you have, in your own way, been developing your courage.

When we are motivated to change something in our lives, or in ourselves, we may often have mixed feelings; for example, some time ago, I made a decision to lose some weight. I was able to connect with a desire to be healthier, to feel more energy and to generally feel better about the way I looked. Still, there was a part of me that was unhappy about this proposed new course of action. My attachment to eating fresh pasta, or homemade chocolate-chip cookies, resulted in some serious mixed feelings about denying myself the chance to eat what I wanted, when I wanted. But mixed feelings are natural, and pretending they aren't swirling around won't help. Ultimately, I found it helpful to make space for the whole range of my feelings about weight loss. I tried to befriend both my ambition to be healthier and my sense of deprivation and entitlement when dieting. The trick was to allow these mixed feelings to be there, without handing my behaviour and my life over to them. As a result, I did wind up losing the weight I'd hoped to, but not without the occasional bit of chocolate or ravioli finding its way into my diet.

To fully realize our compassionate motivation and allow it to flourish, we recognize that our aspiration to care for ourselves may need to share space in our hearts and minds with our anger, our anxiety, our peevishness, and our resistance to, and fear of, change. Rolling with this resistance and opening ourselves to the totality of these different feelings is a necessary part of the awakening of compassionate motivation.

Another key aspect of the compassion circle is *sensitivity*, which means paying attention to the various things that trigger our anxiety, to how anxiety is experienced in our body, sensing the emotions that accompany these physical sensations, and paying attention to the kinds of thoughts that come with the anxiety. Compassionate sensitivity does not just mean that we become increasingly reactive, but that we become increasingly flexible and able to respond as we become more intimately and acutely aware of the quality of how we experience things moment by moment. It means that our attention is more available and open to our difficulties and our response to them. As our compassionate sensitivity grows, we learn how to focus on and notice what anxiety is provoking in us or others.

It's easy to avoid or deny what we are experiencing, especially when we're anxious, but if we're going to be compassionate to ourselves and come to terms with our experience of suffering due to our anxiety, we need to train ourselves to pay attention to the things that may be contributing to our difficulty, and adopt a curious and open point of view.

This training can also help us learn to notice what helps us deal with our anxiety. Of course being out of the anxiety-provoking situation or engaging in various safety-seeking behaviours can temporarily reduce anxiety – but the aim is to 'get better not just feel better'. We can learn to pay attention to things that will help us respond in truly helpful ways – maybe by noting how to breathe soothingly and rhythmically, or maybe by noticing what happens when we change our way of thinking to a more compassionate-minded approach. The more we practise something the more confident we become and it may be useful if you note down the mini-steps you've taken to respond to your anxiety differently, such as when you respond positively to other peoples' smiles or kind words, or feel empowered by meeting new people, or even just one new person, at a party. When you notice what works for you in the face of anxiety, you can build on these things and expand your range of workable, useful responses.

The third attribute of the compassionate mind in the CFT model is described as *sympathy*, and it involves being open to, and directly emotionally touched by, the suffering of others and ourselves. *Compassionate sympathy* is our ability to be emotionally in tune with our anxiety, so we're not running away from it or denying it but instead feel sympathetic towards ourselves, and moved by our distress so that we are motivated to do something about it. Sympathy stands in direct contrast to anger – to getting angry with ourselves or angry with our anxiety. It is the activation of our emotional systems, the way we feel, in response to perceived pain, or even perceived joy in the flourishing of ourselves or someone else. Compassionate sympathy is not the same thing as being frightened of your anxiety or as pitying yourself for your anxiety. It's a kind sensitivity to distress. We have an understanding of how painful and distressing anxiety can be sometimes and just as our heart goes out to others who suffer from anxiety so, too, should we feel sympathetic towards ourselves and our own suffering.

If our compassionate mind training allows us to become increasingly sensitive and sympathetic, it makes a great deal of sense that we would aim to also develop *distress tolerance*, which involves learning how to tolerate our experience of anxiety without thinking we must turn off our feelings or buy into our internal stories that tell us, 'I can't possibly bear this.' Our sensitivity will allow us to notice thoughts and attitudes that might be pushing us away from *compassionate distress tolerance* – and instead give us the feeling that the distress is overwhelming, rather than just deeply unpleasant. In order to experience and adapt our responses to suffering in others and ourselves, we can develop the capacity to tolerate distress and remain in the presence of disturbing feelings without feeling overwhelmed.

Compassionate distress tolerance allows us to experience our internal response to pain and suffering without surrendering our outward behaviour to our distress. Although we may still experience discomfort, worry and fear, we will gradually develop the ability to tolerate these states, and make choices about how we wish to act in the world.

We often wish our anxiety would just go away, and perhaps fantasize that therapy, pills or meditation would immediately banish our apprehension and take us to a state of ongoing bliss. But this isn't how this life tends to unfold, no matter how psychologically minded, wise or productive we might become. It may be a bit disheartening to discover that part of well-being involves learning how to tolerate distress but we can be assured that the compassionate development of resilience, proceeding step by step, will provide us with new ways of responding that allow us to be less frightened, and more able to cope.

There are many times in life where we have to tolerate anxiety; for example, the first time you drove a car, maybe during a driving lesson, was probably rather frightening. Taking a major exam, such as the entrance exam to university, could also be frightening. But despite your fear and anxiety you may have tolerated such feelings because you had an incentive that if you made it through the challenging experience the rewards would be good for you. Notice how this links to the things we explored in the motivation section. Learning distress tolerance helps keep us going in the direction of our valued aims. After all, those things that bring meaning and vitality to our lives are the reasons we are willing to engage with painful feelings. When you pass your driver's test you get freedom to come and go as you please; when you pass your entrance exams you get to further your education and move your life in the direction that brings you fulfilment.

There is no point in tolerating things that are not useful. If you are being pressured by your peers to do something you know is either wrong or that you feel completely uncomfortable with, your compassionate mind will help you to have the courage to say no. Likewise, when there are other aims that you wish to pursue, but which seem difficult, your capacity for distress tolerance becomes an important strength. One of the great costs of anxiety is the degree to which our struggle with it devours our time and energy, and keeps us away from more profound and rewarding activities. Perhaps we avoid job interviews because we fear we will be rejected. Or remain at home engrossed in worries rather than spending time with friends, seeking out new experiences, or building new relationships. Compassionate distress tolerance can help us live fuller lives.

Research has proven that people who have more positive and realistic beliefs about their ability to tolerate emotions are better able to respond flexibly to their experiences both good and bad, are more mindful of the present moment, are better able to make decisions and are less prone to depression and anxiety.[1] In CFT, compassionate distress tolerance affords us the opportunity to experience difficult emotions, and to continue to move towards what matters most to us.

In our CFT model, *empathy* is the attribute of the compassionate mind that involves our capacity to think about, understand and comprehend the suffering we encounter in the world. It relates to how we understand that we and others have motivations, emotions, desires and fantasies that often underpin our behaviour. It relates to our understanding that we and others are products of evolution and desire, and that we feel similar things – we are not alien to each other. Empathy enables us to understand that we, and our values, desires and emotions, are also product of our history, and the sources of our feelings (including anxieties) can be found both in our histories and in the present moment.

The processing of the emotional pain of others and ourselves is known as *compassionate empathy*, and is linked to our ability to tolerate distress. Here's how it works: imagine that somebody tells you that your friend's mother has died. When you ring her she is crying, and still very distressed and grief-stricken. Although you did not know your friend's mother, you are able to appreciate the range and depth of your friend's emotional experience. You can feel her anxiety and grief as if you were experiencing it yourself. Your empathy allows you to imagine what is going through her mind and body. *Compassionate empathy* allows you to recognize what might be helpful to her, how you might hold her in kindness, connect with her through your speech, or offer practical help. Beyond any logical or problem-solving mode, your empathy allows you to sense this experience from her perspective, to feel as she might feel, and to be moved by this awareness. Whereas your sympathy might want you to make it better for her – for the pain to just go away (and that is a compassionate and understandable desire), your empathy helps you understand this is not possible and that what she needs is someone who'll simply listen and who will understand and validate her experience and feelings.

Our empathy provokes a curiosity, and a desire to explore, engage with, and work to alleviate the suffering that we are in intimate contact with. *Compassionate empathy* involves our capacity for gaining perspective, our ability to discern and internally represent the mental experience of others so that we can better understand another's needs, aspirations, emotions and concerns. Related to this is *self-compassionate empathy*, which when directed to yourself does the same thing as you did for your friend. It enables you to think about your anxiety, understand what your anxiety is really about, and what it needs in order to settle. Empathy invites you to react with wisdom and kindness, even if that means simply to understand and validate your feelings.

Another attribute of the CFT model is 'non-judgement', which involves our capacity to view ourselves and others from a non-condemning and non-judgemental perspective. As we have seen, anxiety often involves the activation of shame and self-blame. Depression and other unpleasant states also often involve severe self-criticism, or a hostile and judgemental view of ourselves or others. Our internal critic often keeps a running commentary, judging which feelings are good or bad. But we have seen how the effects of mindfulness involve a suspension of judging and an flexible attention to the present moment. The attribute of *compassionate non-judgement* involves our willingness to experience whatever presents itself without buying into or being ruled by our negative self-judgement, criticism or condemnation. Compassionate non-judgement encourages us to experience our thoughts and feelings for what they are, and allows us to connect with a central theme in CFT – that our thoughts, feelings and behavioural urges are not our fault. Compassionate non-judgement can help us cultivate our compassionate minds.

Indeed, each of the attributes described above represent foundations for the activation of our compassionate minds and these are interdependent, and support each other: if one attribute weakens or lessens then compassion may falter. Imagine compassion without the motivation to be caring and helpful or without the desire to be tolerant of our distress or feel empathy.

With this in mind, sometimes we need to do more work on one attribute than on another. All of them can be expanded and strengthened by compassionate mind training specific to each attribute. The training is designed to proceed gradually, and allow us to shape new behaviours and capacities through small, consistent steps. We can't cram for them, as we would for an exam we hadn't studied for properly, or pull an all-nighter to get the job done. Instead, the process is a gradual one, and takes effort.

Compassionate Skills

Compassionate skills are what we develop when we train our compassionate mind and include motivation, empathy, distress tolerance and so on that, in turn, help us live with, and cope with, our anxiety. Compassionate skills help us develop distress tolerance, styles of thinking that might help us develop empathy and ways to be flexible, calm and capable of interacting with and adapting to our environment. These skills involve learning to focus and activate our compassionate attention in a gentle and flexible way.

Compassionate attention involves directing our awareness to events in our outer and inner environments and relates to the quality, the direction and the object of our attention, which, as we will see, can go a long way to helping us respond to our anxiety. For a moment, let's return to my client Jennifer, and imagine that she is experiencing a rushed and hurried day at school, and is under the pressure of deadlines and faculty politics. She might find herself so caught up in the flow of the demands of the workplace that her field of attention has been narrowed by stress and anxiety and has caused her to attend to negative predictions and hassles. She might be darting her eyes toward the clock and running on autopilot while her threat-detection system runs into the red. In contrast though, let's imagine the same situation with Jennifer skilfully deploying mindful, compassionate attention to what is going on around her. She may still feel anxious and stressed; however, her compassionate attention is allowing her to tune in to her emotional awareness with acceptance and warmth, moment by moment, and in turn allow her to notice some of the more positive and rewarding aspects of her work and reconnect with her purpose of helping to shape the lives of her very young students. Her active, compassionate awareness gives her the breathing room and working space to function more smoothly and calmly, and helps her to take care of herself, as much as she can, throughout the day. This kind of quality and focus of attention emerges as we develop the ability to engage and activate our emotion-regulation system that can access our own place of safety, our own 'affiliation', and provide a sense of acceptance, kindness and a secure base from which to operate. Mindfulness training is an excellent way for us to begin to cultivate compassionate attention in order to better be able to access the calming wisdom of self-compassion.

The second compassionate mind training skill involves our ability to engage in compassionate thinking, whereby we adopt a wider perspective and flow of thoughts in tune with a compassionate way of being. It is important to remember that we aren't pursuing compassion for some abstract reason. All of our work in compassionate mind training is in response to anxiety and is aimed at helping you build a greater sense of well-being and thus the freedom to take your life in the direction you want it to go.

The key questions to ask yourself are: Is the way I'm thinking helpful to me? Is it workable in the long run? Does it give me a wider perspective that opens up opportunities for me, and move me towards my goals and values? Or does my thinking focus on threats, and take me in repetitive cycles where I get more anxious or worrisome and see my options closing down?

Compassionate thinking is when we make a decision to note the kind of thoughts going through our minds, particularly those linked to threats. Then, we make the decision to notice such thoughts as what they are: events in our minds. When we do this we may decide to pause, draw attention into the present moment through an awareness of our breathing and ask ourselves if we need to buy into and surrender to our threatened-mind thinking, or if there may be a more workable, purposeful and compassionate way to respond to our environment in the here and now.

Granted, sometimes it may be helpful to be accurate and clear about what's guiding our thinking; for example, if your anxiety involves fear of having a heart attack then it's important to get the information about the difference between feelings of panic and the true signs a cardiac arrest. However, compassion is key – you're directing your thinking to be helpful, and it may not be helpful to seek evidence for the accuracy or veracity of our fears. In fact, I've worked with many clients who have obsessively poured over the Internet to search for data about how likely it would be for them to die in a plane crash, or become ill from microwave-oven radiation. The data only serves to stir up their anxiety. Sometimes 'looking for the evidence' can get us caught in a loop of safety-seeking behaviour that activates our threat-detection system and bounces us around on waves of fear and apprehension. Additionally, sometimes highly accurate thoughts might not be very useful in a given situation. We can revisit the example of trying to escape from a high floor of a burning building by climbing down the fire escape: it might be accurate to think that 'If I fall I will die', nevertheless, although this is true, it isn't going to help you make your way down. Instead, if you focus on making your way down the fire escape, albeit clinging on for dear life, you can also then focus on your grip and your footholds and carefully as you can as you ease your way down. This is a good example of what we mean by compassionate thinking, which comes from a position of encouragement, warmth, kindness and understanding rather than from cold logic. Remember that the definition of compassion involves recognition of your anxiety and suffering, and an aspiration to do something about it.

Sometimes people can be very good at recognizing that their anxiety is irrational; however, they might look at the evidence and then think, 'My heart is racing and it's scaring me but I'm fit and healthy and am not about to have a heart attack. I'm being stupid to be frightened.' Here, being able to discern that you are experiencing anxiety rather than having a heart attack might give you a bit of relief, but the tone of condemnation and the desire to suppress the thoughts might actually be counterproductive. Unleashing your inner critic and trying to avoid your fears might have a semblance of rationality to it, but may be unlikely to help you deal with your threatened-mind mode. In fact, as you angrily tell yourself off, you might even stoke up the activity of your fight-or-flight response by becoming irritable at perceived threats. Alternatively, if you access your compassionate mind, and your compassionate thinking, you can be more patient and understanding towards yourself and your fears. You can encourage yourself to face the fear, let it wash over you and then shift your focus to other, more positive things. Time and again we come back to this motivation to be helpful. The aim is to be supportive, whether it's by generating alternate, more positive thoughts, by becoming better able to adapt to our thought processes or by allowing ourselves to be exposed to the things that scare us.

From this foundation of compassionate attention and compassionate thinking we are free to engage in compassionate behaviour that embodies our awareness of suffering, and our desire to alleviate suffering. Such compassionate behaviour allows us bear our anxiety with warmth and self-kindness, as we move towards living our lives fully, with purpose and vitality. Compassion is not about being nice to ourselves in an indulgent way but in a 'moving forward' way. If you are agoraphobic, you might find that you are more comfortable sitting at home but that may be far from compassionate behaviour towards yourself. Compassionate behaviour is finding the courage to make a commitment to engage with and overcome your anxiety by going out.

Compassionate behaviour helps us face up to possible feelings of shame when we choose to seek help if our anxiety seems too much or if we are depressed. Remember, this book is not an alternative to therapy and if you are feeling depressed or overwhelmed by your anxiety I would encourage you to seek professional help. Compassionate behaviour is very much about opening ourselves to others and allowing ourselves to be helped. Compassionate behaviour *is not* about struggling on by ourselves when help could make it so much easier. Although I will be talking about bearing anxiety and living with it in the present moment, compassionate behaviour is not being overwhelmed and masochistically tolerating pain. Whatever steps you take, do it in the spirit of helpfulness to you, with the aim of *developing* yourself *step by step* and getting what help you need as you go.

Compassionate behaviour involves caring for ourselves, such as by establishing regular patterns of sleeping and waking, or maintaining a healthy and nourishing diet, of engaging in regular exercise, or physical activities that promote health and release of tension. Sometimes, though, compassionate behaviour may not seem to be something we typically associate with compassion. For example, gathering up the courage to attend an anxiety-provoking meeting because it is important for your professional development may be a form of compassionate behaviour. It may repeatedly involve acts of courage and resolve. For example, a parent who is anxious about their teenage child's problems with drugs and alcohol may need to summon the courage to compassionately confront their child, and aim to organize treatment for the problems. When we engage in compassionate behaviour we are consciously taking care of ourselves, even though it may seem distressing at the time. When we cultivate our compassionate mind, we are activating and developing an ancient social mentality that has been designed by evolution to allow us to feel strong and calm, even when we are in the midst of anxiety and a sense of danger.

Our circle diagram includes a few other skills that combine with attention, thinking and behaviour to round out the capacities involved in compassionate mind training: *compassionate sensory processing* involves using our awareness to contact physical sensations in a non-judgemental, open and self-compassionate way. This involves learning how to breathe regularly and smoothly (we'll learn about this in Part II) and to hold the body in ways that allow you to engage with your anxiety with willingness, mindfulness and self-kindness. Elements of compassionate sensory processing will be used for some of our imagery-based exercises. As we will discover, connecting specific sensory experiences to our experience of the compassionate mind, such as feeling our facial muscles forming a warm, gently smiling expression, can be helpful in activating our compassion and mindfulness and soothing our anxiety. *Compassionate imagery* is how we create images in our minds that will stimulate the affiliative, supportive system that fuels and sustains our compassionate mind. If, for example, we allowed our mind to brew up a stream of disturbing, frightening images, and allowed ourselves to be so immersed in such images that they begin to dominate our behaviour, we run the risk of handing our lives over to the domination of our threat-detection system and our threatened mind. If, on the other hand, we deliberately practise focusing on compassionate images such as nurturing figures, who accept us and provide us with a safe and soothing place, or images of being compassionate to ourselves, we may be able to activate our compassionate mind, and begin to manage our anxiety. Developing the skill of compassionate imagery can take some time, and can be challenging; however, steady, gradual work in this area may begin to offer us new ways of engaging with, and freeing ourselves from, excessive experiences of anxiety.

A lot of these skills might not seem specific to training our compassionate minds, and are often a part of our everyday experiences. We are often moved to help others, to be supportive and kind. The 'skilfulness' we are seeking to cultivate in compassionate mind training involves bringing these qualities to life in ourselves, and in response to the suffering we encounter ourselves over the course of our lives. The aim is to activate our compassionate mind as we need it, moment by moment, in response to the challenges of life.

Remember that it is our intentions that are important – even if we do not have certain feelings. Sometimes warmth is hard to muster but it is worth trying to be kind and compassionate even if we do not feel it – feelings can come later – with practice. We may try to be kind to our family even if we are in a bad mood and don't feel like it! Nonetheless an important element of all of the above, both attributes and skills, is to cultivate and generate feelings of warmth and kindness. This is where some people can begin to struggle. They may say they can feel kindness for others but cannot feel it for themselves. This is common. We know that when we are distressed those feeling systems may not be working quite so well, so it's only natural if we struggle to feel warmly towards ourselves. We might have to wait for that system to get going a bit and the best way to do this is to practise compassionate attention, thinking and behaviour, and allow the feelings to follow with time.

As we begin to function in more compassionate ways, perhaps even to extend our hearts and hands towards others, our minds become more sensitive to both our own emotions and the emotions of others. We may become better able to notice and discern the quality of our own anxiety, and the anxiety of those around us, without this anxiety feeling as if it may be a catastrophe in and of itself. When we are intimately in contact with our own experience, moment by moment, we may be willing to experience life just as it presents itself, which may include the present-ation of our anxious feelings and thoughts.

Part II

Compassionate Mind Training for Anxiety

6 Mindfulness as a Foundation for Compassionate Attention

> The brain can only assume its proper behaviour when consciousness is doing what it is designed for: not writhing and whirling to get out of present experience, but being effortlessly aware of it.
>
> Alan Watts, *The Wisdom of Insecurity*[1]

At the beginning of this book, I had said that if you were holding this book, you probably had some experience with anxiety. Well, if you have read this far, then you also may have begun to understand something about self-compassion and the motivation to overcome problems with anxiety. I'm glad that you have let yourself take the time to explore how our evolutionary origins have led us to possess a capacity for self-compassion that can help us to experience calmness, flexibility and courage, even in the presence of anxiety. We now can capitalize on what you have learned so far and begin to directly engage in compassionate mind training, using the techniques of CFT.

Mindfulness

Jon Kabat-Zinn famously defined mindfulness as 'the kind of awareness that emerges from paying attention in a particular way: on purpose, in the present moment, and non-judgementally'.[2] It is something that is better understood through experience than by explanation: imagine how much more you could learn about swimming by being in the water than by reading about the backstroke. Nevertheless, mindfulness can easily be experienced by practising some fundamental exercises that work with our attention, moment by moment. We will begin looking at some of these exercises shortly; however, mindful awareness is far more than just a practised method of meditation and the aim is for it to become a way of being that allows us to encounter each experience with a growing degree of openness, acceptance and self-compassion.

Over the past several years, mindfulness training has become an increasingly popular and important part of Western therapy and a great deal of the emphasis on the benefits of mindfulness training has involved helping people deal with anxiety-related stress, which is, as we discussed earlier, linked to the activation of our threatened minds. So, it makes sense that we begin with mindfulness when we begin to train ourselves to develop our compassionate response to anxiety.

For just a moment, let's look a little bit closer at the origins of practising mindfulness. While much traditional wisdom uses attention-training exercises that resemble what we call mindfulness, the CFT concept of mindfulness is derived from the methods of the Buddha. The Sanskrit term that is now translated into English as 'mindfulness' was 'sati', which describes a particular, deliberate way of paying attention that involves a blend of present-moment-focused attention, open awareness, and memory of oneself.[3] Sati wasn't pursued as an end unto itself but was used as a way of deliberately opening and shifting awareness to promote more healthy and 'wholesome' states of mind, such as the state of being compassionate and wise.[4] According to the Buddha, training in sati was important for overcoming anxious and apprehensive states of mind.

Directly Learning about Attention

Despite what we are learning about mindfulness, it is important to remember that it is ultimately an *experiential* process, in other words: we learn by doing it. So, let's begin with an attention-training exercise that will prepare the way for our mindfulness practice.

This first exercise can be viewed as a game or experiment that can teach us about the nature of attention. It doesn't take a great deal of time, or a whole lot of effort.

To begin, sit quietly for a moment and concentrate on your left foot.

Notice the feeling in your toes, and the soles of the feet. Then, after about twenty seconds, switch your concentration on to your right foot, noticing the sensations that are present in the heel and toes and so on. Then, again about twenty seconds later, bring your attention to your fingers by gently rubbing your thumbs over your fingertips.

Take a moment and then with your next natural exhale let this part of the exercise go.

What happened to your awareness of your fingers when you were focusing on your left foot? What happened to the awareness of your right foot when you were focusing on your fingers? You have just noticed that what you pay attention to becomes larger in your mind than other things you were previously paying attention to and which fade from your mind as you redirect your attention.

Our attention, then, helps us to focus our awareness, and acts like a sort of zoom lens that brings into focus one particular thing at a time.

Here is another exercise: sit quietly for a minute and simply remember a time when you were happy, when somebody made you really laugh, when you heard a funny joke or when you were outside enjoying the sunshine on a beautiful spring day. Remember it in as much detail as you can. How did you feel? Who was with you? Notice what happens to your feelings as you focus your attention on this memory; notice how you may even want to smile again.

OK, now take a breath and bring something new to mind: for just a few moments recall a time when you were upset. Recall what was happening around you but don't stay in that memory for too long. Notice what happened in your body, and what happened to those happy feelings. Did you feel differently when your attention was directed towards something new?

The changes in your feelings highlight the idea that your attention influences our feelings, and that you can learn to take notice of, and direct the focus of your attention, *yourself*.

This brief exercise has demonstrated that our attention can, to some degree, be *moved around voluntarily*. Though our attention rarely stays put, if we remember our aim, we can return our attention again and again towards a certain orientation.

The exercise has also made us aware of the way the direction of our attention affects the way we feel, both physically and mentally and it is useful to understand this when we begin to deal with our anxiety. We can work with our attention, and learn how to do this by practising the next few practical exercises that will help us connect our attention to the fundamentals of mindfulness.

Soothing-Rhythm Breathing

For our first exercise, we will begin by focusing on the natural rhythm of our breathing, allowing our breath to find its own pace and calming rhythm.

Instructions

As we begin our exercises, please find a comfortable place to sit where you can keep both feet on the floor, and can allow your back to be straight. Your spine should not be rigid, but supple and straight, in a posture described by CFT practitioners as 'dignified' or 'grounded'. Allow your feet to rest approximately shoulders' width apart and allow your arms to be relaxed and hanging gently, with your hands resting lightly on the top of your thighs. Make any small adjustments to your posture as we begin, and feel free to make such adjustments later if you need. As much as you can, allow yourself to fall silent and still but allow yourself to feel comfortable and settled rather than trying to rigidly hold on to any particular posture. Now, allow your eyes to close, and draw your attention to the gentle flow of your breath in and out of the body. Feel your connection to your breath as it moves within you and when it is released. Continue to focus on your breath without aiming to change or correct anything at all; simply breathe in, and out.

After a moment, direct your attention to the flow of your breath, feeling it fill your belly as if there were a balloon in your abdomen that gently expands with air as you inhale, and then collapses as you exhale. Feel your diaphragm muscles stretch and your ribcage grow rounder as you inhale, and then feel the muscles push in and the ribcage contract as you exhale.

Notice next the movement of your belly, as it expands and contracts, yet all the while allow your breath to find its own rhythm and its own pace. You may notice the experience of the breath going slightly faster or slightly slower. If so, experiment with this for a moment, and ultimately allow the breath to be where it is, and how it wishes to be. In this way, your breath is giving way to its own soothing rhythm, moment by moment. With each inhale, connect with the sensation of breathing in; with each exhale, connect with the sensation of breathing out. Allow your breath to gradually slow down, and with each natural exhale draw your attention to the sensation of letting go with the whole body.

Most often, our breath becomes somewhat slower and steadier during this practice. It may be helpful to feel the in-breath for a count of three seconds, holding for a moment, and then releasing with the out-breath for a count of three seconds. Taking special care, notice the fullness of the experience of the out-breath.

For a little while, remain attendant to the soothing rhythm of your breath: feel it descending through the diaphragm and into the belly, notice the rising and falling of the abdomen, and sense the release of the exhalation. With part of your attention on the flow of your breath, bring some attention now to your feet on the floor, to your legs on the chair, to your back feeling straight and supported, and to the top of your head. Notice the sensation of being grounded and supported in your posture and, through your feet, being connected and rooted to the Earth. All the while, the soothing rhythm of your breathing continues, as you follow it with gentle, supportive attention.

During this practice, inevitably, your mind will wander. This is perfectly OK and, indeed, a necessary part of our practice. Take a moment to kindly give yourself some credit for noticing that your mind has wandered and gently return your attention to the breath with the next inhalation. This process of gently noticing where the mind is in the present moment and then gently returning awareness to the breath through the inhalation is at the heart of cultivating mindfulness through soothing-rhythm breathing. No matter how often your mind may wander, simply notice wherever it has gone, then draw your attention back into the body with the next natural inhale. When you notice that your mind has wandered, you are noticing the very nature of the mind, and observing that it moves in waves. It is the nature of the mind to wander, and it is the nature of our mindfulness practice to gently and non-judgementally guide our attention back to the flow of the breath.

After a short while practising this soothing-rhythm breathing, allow yourself to exhale and let go of the exercise entirely. Before you open your eyes, give yourself some credit for having engaged with this exercise, and recognize that you have taken some very important time to devote attention solely to yourself, as part of a process of cultivating well-being. When you are ready, open your eyes and return to your everyday awareness.[5]

Reflecting upon Your First Mindfulness Practice

If you were to begin learning mindfulness exercises with a therapist or meditation instructor, you might follow your first experience of soothing-rhythm breathing with a conversation. With your teacher's guidance, you would have the opportunity to take the time to reflect and share some of your observations. Since you are learning these practices from this book, and may be working on your own, it will be helpful for you to ask these questions of yourself, and for yourself. To encourage you to make some space for your experience, and to notice any observations that may be presenting themselves to you, a number of questions are listed below. Please take a few moments to look at these questions, and to respond. When you are done, take some time to review your observations.

As we move forward, and as you begin to practise mindfulness, it would be a good idea to record your observations.

Questions to Ask Yourself after Your
First Soothing-Rhythm Breathing Practice

1. What did you notice about your thoughts, feelings, and physical sensations as you engaged in this exercise?

2. How was the attention you experienced during the soothing-rythm breathing different from your everyday, typical way of paying attention?

3. How might soothing-rhythm breathing help you deal with your anxiety?

4. Were there any obstacles or difficulties that presented themselves as you practised the soothing-rhythm breathing exercise?

5. How might you bring some of the quality of mindfulness that you experienced in this first exercise to an everyday activity, such as washing up, or making a cup of tea?

How to Practice

Mindfulness is a quality of attention that requires regular practice; for example, if I hired a personal trainer, and went to the gym for one session, this probably wouldn't change the way I look, would it? Likewise, if I planted a sapling it wouldn't become shady tree overnight. Lots of things take time to grow, and mindfulness is one of them. But evidence shows that, if practised regularly, mindfulness meditation can significantly reduce anxiety, improve our immune function and change our brain activity in as little as eight weeks.[6] Beyond mindfulness, our training to cultivate our compassionate mind will involve some form of regular practice and it's a good idea to begin by committing to setting aside a small amount of time each day for this purpose. It may vary from week to week, but commitment of some time and some consistency of effort will be of great benefit.

Typically, it is a good idea to begin to practise mindfulness daily for at least the first few weeks. This would serve as a good foundation for building your compassionate attention. I know that it might seem daunting at first, but beginning in this way is an act of self-kindness and self-compassion that can have gradual, but profoundly positive effect on your anxiety. Regardless, it is important to start where you are, and practice however you can. Some of the practical exercises we will look at can take as little as three minutes, and when you become more practised you will find that you will be able to bring compassionate and mindful attention to your state of being in the space of a single breath. Our work in CFT involves a gradual, gentle approach to the cultivation of your capacity of mindful self-compassion, so it is useful to think about what you can aim for, to observe your experience moment by moment, day by day, and week by week as you continue to practise.

As you read through these instructions, aim to recall the central ideas and steps they involve, and then engage in the practice on your own. People often find it helpful to begin mindfulness training with an audio guide. If you wish, you can download audio examples of similar exercises from my website www.mindfulcompassion.com and you can listen to these by using your computer or mp3 player.

Where to Practice

It would be a good idea to establish a regular setting where you can return to easily enter into and begin each exercise. This may be a quiet place in your home, or even your office, where you are most likely be free from interruption. It doesn't have to be anywhere special, spiritual or religious, but it does help if it is somewhere that feels safe, and a space that you can devote solely to yourself, with a compassionate intention for your own well-being.

For a number of exercises, you will be sitting with your back straight and supported for a period of several minutes and it would be good if you could find a comfortable chair, or even a cushion designed for meditation. It might also be helpful to devote some care to how your space looks and feels. Many people who regularly practise mindfulness and compassion-ate mind training will pay close attention to the cleanliness and the beauty of the space they devote to meditation and practice. When such a space is free from clutter and feels organized it can be a mirror to the clarity that we seek. Sometimes, people find it helpful to display images or personal items that embody compassion, or which they find pleasant. These can be sym-bolic items, such as a picture that has special meaning or a beautiful feather you found when you were on a walk. People who meditate under spiritual traditions such as Buddhism, Hinduism or Christianity may choose sym-bols from their faiths that remind them of ideas like forgiveness, acceptance or loving kindness; however, despite drawing on some Buddhist ideas, our practice requires nothing with any spiritual association.

Overall, the aim is to allow yourself to take just a little time to set aside a space that feels like the right environment for you to pursue a greater sense of well-being, contentment and calm.

As you cultivate compassionate attention you may encounter some anxiety-provoking experiences and some people find that the safe envir-onment they've created for their mindful meditation can help them feel safe and supported.

When to Practice

It might not be surprising that many of us find it difficult to squeeze even a fifteen-minute mindfulness exercise into our heavily scheduled, demanding days. Many of the clients I've worked with over the years have found it challenging to develop a consistent mindfulness practice because it is 'so hard to find the time'. In my experience, this can be particularly challenging for people who experience high levels of anxiety, and often worry that if they set aside some time for the development of their own mindfulness and self-care, they will be overlooking something else that is 'very important'. All too frequently, people who are struggling with feelings of shame and anxiety, and who are striving to prove that they are 'good enough', find it challenging to set aside time for themselves. Remember, though, that making the decision to cultivate mindfulness and learning to begin to move towards the development of the compassionate mind is, in itself, an act of self-compassion. It can give us a place to rest in the present moment, and activate our experience of a secure, safe and stable relationship with ourselves.

Establishing a regular time for practice and, as much as we can, returning to the practice with reliability and consistency can be important to our growth and it can be rewarding. Beginning the day with mindfulness practice can set the tone for the rest of the day by turning our minds and attention towards a non-judgemental, open and receptive experience of the present moment. For this reason, I often recommend that mindfulness be scheduled as a part of the morning routine. When we have lived with chronic anxiety and worry, mornings are often the time of day when we begin the struggle with our anxious thoughts and emotions; however, although mindfulness training is particularly well suited for a morning practice, it is more important that we establish regularity, and find a time of day that will work best for us. It is more important to have consistent practice than to schedule your practice at a particular time of day that may not suit you. Generally speaking, even five minutes of formal mindfulness training on a daily basis will be more beneficial than longer periods of irregular practice.

Recording your daily practice, the times when you've engaged in mindfulness training and whatever observations you might have, can really support and sustain your work. I've included a form below, so that you can follow your progress, structure your work and reflect upon what you have learned, day by day, and week by week. You can use this form for any of the mindfulness practices we will be looking at.

My Mindfulness Practice Record		
Date	*Daily Practice*	*What did you notice?*
Monday Date: Length of time in practice:	Any mindfulness practice today? (Yes or No) If you practised, did you use an audio guide? (Yes or No)	
Tuesday Date: Length of time in practice:	Any mindfulness practice today? (Yes or No) If you practised, did you use an audio guide? (Yes or No)	
Wednesday Date: Length of time in practice:	Any mindfulness practice today? (Yes or No) If you practised, did you use an audio guide? (Yes or No)	
Thursday Date: Length of time in practice:	Any mindfulness practice today? (Yes or No) If you practised, did you use an audio guide? (Yes or No)	
Friday Date: Length of time in practice:	Any mindfulness practice today? (Yes or No) If you practised, did you use an audio guide? (Yes or No)	
Saturday Date: Length of time in practice:	Any mindfulness practice today? (Yes or No) If you practised, did you use an audio guide? (Yes or No)	
Sunday Date: Length of time in practice:	Any mindfulness practice today? (Yes or No) If you practised, did you use an audio guide? (Yes or No)	

Further Mindfulness Exercises

In CFT, mindfulness training typically begins with soothing-rhythm breathing but there are a range of other mindfulness practices that can prepare us to access and activate self-compassion in response to our anxiety, worry and fear. The following practical exercises may be used regularly to cultivate mindful awareness. I would recommend that you choose one exercise for a given one- to three-week period to give yourself the chance to explore and deepen your practice of this exercise before moving on to another.

The Body Scan

When anxiety arrives, we notice it in our thoughts, our emotional reactions and also in our physical sensations; however, by bringing mindful awareness to the body, we can change our relationship to our anxious physical sensations, and respond with greater flexibility and temper the activation of our threat-detection system.

The Body Scan is an exercise that many people find particularly effective for calmly and restfully dealing with stress, and it is well suited to help us learn to work with anxiety using our attention. It helps us direct a mindful, non-judgemental awareness of the body at a gradual and deliberate pace. The directions below will guide you through the process.

Instructions

The exercise is usually conducted lying down, or seated with the back straight yet supple. It would be best if you found a comfortable space and used a yoga mat, rug or blanket to lie on. The temperature should also be comfortable and the exercise at time when you will be free from distraction or interruption.

To begin, let your eyes close, and allow yourself to rest but not sleep. Allow yourself to fall silent and still. Gently direct your attention to the physical sensations you are experiencing and bring your attention to the presence of life in the body.

Allow yourself to observe the flow of your breath, as it moves gently in and out of your body. There is no need to breathe in any special way; just allow the breath to find its own rhythm. As you breathe in, notice the physical sensations involved in the inhalation. When you release the breath, allow your attention to flow out with the exhalation.

With each in-breath, gather and collect attention, and with each out-breath let go of that awareness.

Now, gently direct your attention to the physical sensations you are experiencing throughout your body at this moment. With each inhalation, allow your attention to gather at the contact points where your body meets the mat, the chair or the cushion that supports you, and feel your weight sinking into them. As you exhale, noticing the heaviness you feel as your weight seems to sink further.

There is no need to aim for any special state of being during this practice. There is no need to strive to relax, or to do anything at all but simply observe what you are experiencing moment by moment. Let go of the urge to judge, analyse or even describe your experience, and then begin to direct your attention to the different parts of your body.

With the next natural inhale, allow your attention to move to the physical sensations in the abdomen. Notice the various sensations that accompany each in-breath and out-breath. After staying with this experience for a few seconds, bring your attention up from your abdomen, along the length of your left arm, and into the left hand. Allow your attention to spread, as if it were a warm presence radiating down the arm, all the while noticing the presence of life in the body.

Merely observe the sensations in the hand. With each inhale, allow yourself to imagine the breath flowing into the chest and abdomen, and radiating down the left arm into the hand. Your attention will accompany this inhalation, as if you were 'breathing in' awareness of the physical sensations present in the hand. Allow yourself to breathe in to the sensations in each part of the hand for several seconds. With each exhale, allow yourself to let go of that awareness.

As you do this, allow yourself to notice the thumb . . . the index finger . . . the second finger . . . the ring finger . . . and the pinky. Next, breathe in a collected awareness of the sensations in the back of the hand . . . the palm of the hand . . . and the hand as a whole. When you feel that you have completed your gentle observation of the sensations in the left hand, allow your attention to radiate back up the left arm, noticing the presence of life in the lower arm, the bicep, the tricep, and all of the parts of the arm.

With the next natural inhale, allow your attention to gather again in the abdomen. Next, allow yourself to bring this attention to the sensations in the right arm and hand, in the same manner that you used with your left.

At a comfortable pace, and with an attitude of gentle, non-judgemental curiosity, direct your attention to each of the areas of the body in turn. Take your time and spend as long as you need, before exhaling and letting go of this area and moving the attention to the next part of the body. Breathe in to the sensations in each foot (and each of the toes) . . . each lower leg . . . shin . . . and calf . . . the pelvic region . . . the lower back and abdomen . . . the upper back and shoulders . . . the neck . . . and the contact point between the head and the spine, just behind the eyes . . . now, bring attention to the muscles of the face . . . the forehead . . . and the scalp.

Allow yourself to take this slowly and when you observe discomfort or tension in any part of the body, allow yourself to again breathe in to the sensations. As much as you can, attempt to stay with each sensation, merely observing it, being with it moment by moment. Remember that it is the nature of our minds to wander. When you notice that your mind has drifted away from the focus on physical sensations, accept that this has happened, allow some room for this experience in your awareness, and gently draw your attention back to the physical sensations with the next natural inhale.

After you have spent some time engaged in this practice, having brought a mindful awareness to the body over the course of several minutes (this practice can range from fifteen to forty-five or so minutes) gently allow your breath and attention to return to settle on the physical sensations in the abdomen.

Now, with the next natural inhale, allow your attention to focus on the sounds that surround you in the room, then to the sounds outside the room. Following this, allow your attention to gently settle on the sounds even farther away than that. Giving yourself a few moments to gather your attention and orientation to your presence in the room, you can open your eyes, and resume your daily activities.[7]

The Body Scan is a useful practice to engage in regularly for a period of at least two weeks, in order to begin to experience the effect of regular, mindful release of tension, and the direction of flexible, focused, and non-judgemental attention to our experience of stress and anxiety in the body. You can use the log in the last section of this book to record your practice of The Body Scan.

Soften, Soothe and Allow [8]

The Soften, Soothe and Allow exercise is one that many of my patients have benefitted from as a daily practice. It helps us see how we can use mindfulness to make space for our experience of anxiety, and how we might apply mindful and compassionate attention to our experience of distress.

Instructions

Just as we have with our other mindfulness and compassionate-attention exercises, we begin this one by adopting a stable and grounded posture, with the back straight and supported. Settle upon your cushion or chair and allow your breath to settle into the natural pace and rhythm that emerges through your soothing-rhythm breathing. When you are ready, take three more breaths in this way, feeling the release of tension each time you exhale.

With the next natural inhale, direct part of your attention to the sensations that are present in the body. Whatever you notice, allow yourself to continue to focus also on the breath, feeling the movement of the belly, and bring open, non-judgemental attention to the presence of the breath in the area of your heart.

With each inhale, bring compassionate attention into the body, and with each exhale let go of tension, and pay attention to any experience of emotions in the body. What physical sensations, in this moment, feel related to your emotions? Perhaps you have experienced anxiety or distress; if so, this is the time to allow yourself to feel where this emotional experience presents itself as a physical sensation. You may feel anxiety as tension in the chest or throat, for example. Wherever it is, notice it, and bring compassionate attention to this place with each inhale, and feel yourself softening into that space in the body. Imagine this to be similar to applying warmth to stiff or sore muscles. Let go of physically forcing anything at all and repeat the word 'soft' over and over again, with the soothing rhythm of the breath. We aren't aiming to suppress or avoid any experience at all here; we are simply bringing mindful and compassionate attention to our emotional and physical experience in this very moment. Stay with this process of softening for a few minutes.

Having softened into this experience, now, if you would like, bring one of your hands to your chest, just over your heart. Feel the warmth of your hand, and through it direct kindness and soothing thoughts to yourself. Recognize your struggle, and direct warmth and self-acceptance towards yourself and your experience. Speak kindly to yourself, out loud or in your thoughts, validate your struggle with anxiety and distress, and connect with your compassionate inner voice. You may say something like, 'I can see how hard this has been for me now. This pain and these difficult experiences are a part of life, and this is not my fault. May I grow into greater well-being, peacefulness and happiness, moment by moment.'

Next, gently repeat the word 'soothe' in your mind, with part of your attention resting in the soothing rhythm of the breath. You may also choose to imagine the experience of soothing and kindness arriving at that place in the body where you have felt your emotion physically affect you. Notice your inhale and exhale and as much as you can. Remain with this process of soothing for a few more minutes.

As a final step, consciously let go of the need or urge to get rid of your emotional experience. As you exhale let go of any effort to avoid or suppress your emotion. Having softened into the experience, and brought soothing attention to your struggle, ask yourself to allow your discomfort to be just as it is in this moment. The feeling doesn't need to be pushed away. You are in a safe place, and you can just allow this emotion to be where it is, and for it to come and go in its own time. This time, silently repeat the word 'allow' in time with the soothing rhythm of your breath. Just as we have with each gentle step of this practice, stay with this for a few minutes, or however long it feels right to you.

You may choose to silently repeat the words 'soften, soothe, allow' in your mind as your follow the breath during the last minutes of the exercise. Stay with the breath for as long as you need, resting in the soothing rhythm, and directing mindful, compassionate attention to your emotion.

When you are ready, take one last inhale and then exhale slowly and let go of this exercise altogether, giving yourself credit for having deeply engaged with this practice.

Like our earlier mindfulness exercises, Soften, Soothe and Allow can be used daily for a period of several days, weeks or months. This practice, however, may also be used in an abbreviated form to bring compassionate attention into contact with anxiety in the moment it appears to you, wherever you are. This will represent an important transition point, where your practice of mindful awareness begins to move from the meditation cushion to your day-to-day emotion-regulation responses. Our next exercises will take this application of mindfulness skills further into the flow of our everyday life.

The Three-Minute Breathing Space

Soften, Soothe and Allow, the last exercise we looked at, can be used to bring soothing, compassionate and mindful attention to our experiences of stress and anxiety. This next exercise, The Three-Minute Breathing Space, is designed to help us accomplish just that, and can be used when we feel anxiety begin to take hold of us. As the name implies, this exercise is designed to involve a very small time commitment, but that small amount of time can bring enormous benefits, and help us become calm when we begin to suffer from anxiety.

Instructions

The Three-Minute Breathing Space exercise is best begun in a seated position with the soles of your feet touching the ground and your back upright yet supported and comfortable. The aim is to practise the exercise seated but then to be able to engage with the exercise while standing. It is designed to help you breathe life into your mindfulness practice by applying it directly in the flow of your everyday life.

To begin, allow yourself to make any adjustments to your seated posture that may be necessary so that you might sit with a dignified, erect yet relaxed manner. The back is straight. The sit-bones are supported. You can feel yourself rooted to the earth at the contact points where your body meets your chair and the floor. Allow your eyes to close or, if you prefer, just allow the eyelids to relax as you cast your gaze gently at the floor. Now, direct part of your attention to the soles of the feet and then to the flow of experience that unfolds in your mind. Observing thoughts, feelings and physical sensations, allow yourself to notice, as much as you can, what is presenting itself to you at this moment and pay particular attention to those feelings, ideas and sensations that may be unpleasant or upsetting. Rather than pushing these away, allow them to be just as they are. Take a moment, and allow yourself to simply acknowledge the presence of these experiences, making space for whatever emerges and flows through your field of inner observation.

Now, having allowed yourself to sit in the presence of this moment, with whatever it brings, it is time to change your focus and attention towards a single object. Observe your breathing, and direct your attention to the movements of your body as you exhale and inhale. Take special notice of the bellows-like movement of the abdomen, as our body gently allows the air to move in and out, moment by moment. Take a minute to stay with the flow of the breath and allow your attention to blend with the movement of breathing itself, as best as you can.

Next, bring your attention to a third step: allow the scope of your awareness to widen to gradually encompass the entire body. Bring your attention into the body as a whole as you inhale and sense the body gently expanding as you inhale; as you exhale, completely let go of that awareness. Stay with this experience for about a minute, and allow yourself to make space within your body and mind, as best as you can, for whatever arrives.

Next, begin to let go of this exercise, by again directing part of your attention to the soles of your feet, then to the top of your head, and then part of your attention to everything in between. When you are ready, allow your eyes to open and let go of this exercise entirely.[9]

If possible, make time to practise The Three-Minute Breathing Space several times a day, in addition to a daily, regular mindfulness practice such as Soften, Soothe and Allow or The Body Scan. This combination of exercises will allow you to begin your day by focusing on compassionate attention, and then to continue throughout the day to dip into regular mindfulness practice. Additionally, this brief Three-Minute Breathing Space can be used as a coping response during those moments when you feel the intensification of stress and anxiety.

Mindful Walking

As we have learned, mindfulness is more than just a technique that we use to address our problems. It is a natural, human state of being that can allow us to more fully experience the richness of the present moment. As such, our aim is to gradually bring this state of mindful acceptance into our everyday life. We begin with specific practices lying or sitting, and then transition towards taking mindful actions. A good place to begin this transition is with the simple act of walking. The following exercise will guide you through a practice of mindful walking that can be used formally, or informally, so that you might better integrate mindfulness into all of your activities.

Instructions

Find a place, inside or outside, where you may walk for some time with relatively little concern for onlookers or interruptions. You may choose a park, a city block, a shopping mall or even a path through the rooms of your home. Begin by standing with your feet slightly less than shoulders' width apart. Keep your knees supple, your back straight and your arms relaxed. Gaze forward but with a wide-angle focus. As you inhale, direct your attention at the soles of your feet. Allow yourself to sense the connection between your feet and the floor. With each inhale, allow your attention to observe the presence of life in your legs and feet, feeling the distribution of your weight throughout your body; then, with each exhale, let go of this awareness. After some time experiencing this, allow your weight to transfer to the right leg, taking note of all of the richness of the sensations involved. Next, allow yourself to draw your attention to the left leg and transfer your weight. You may experience a sensation of the right leg feeling lighter or 'emptying' as you rely upon it less for support. Allow your attention now to be divided between the legs, noticing the different sensations present throughout your lower body.

When you are ready allow the left foot to slightly lift away from the floor. Notice the sensations in your muscles as it lifts and then gently moves forward to take a first step. Gradually and deliberately move the left leg forward, all the while gently observing the physical sensations that accompany this action. As you complete this first step, notice the sensations involved as you place the left foot back on the floor. Feel the weight transfer as your body uses the leg and foot for support and as its contact with the ground grows heavier and more assured. As this occurs, notice whatever sensations emerge in the right leg as it lets go of the weight and support, growing lighter as the movement continues. As your weight is transferred to the left foot in a stable fashion, repeat this process with the right foot. Breathe into the sensation of the right foot leaving the floor. Observe the presence of life in the body as the right foot moves forward to take your next step. Again, notice the physical sensations as this right foot makes contact with the ground, and you complete this next step. As you do this, allow your motion to flow from one step to the next, rather than complete these steps as discrete, robotic movements. Notice how your intention guides your body, drawing it forward slowly in space and time. Your movements may appear as if they are happening in slow motion. Continue to take these steps in this fashion, continuing along the path that you have chosen. As you do this, keep some of your attention connected to the flow of your breath, and the spreading sensations throughout the body. As you walk, connect your attention to the presence of life throughout your body, noticing with kindness and gentle acceptance any sensations that present themselves. Keep your gaze softly focused ahead of you, aware of your surroundings, but also persistently aware of your presence in your body. As with earlier practices, the mind will inevitably wander from the attention to the act of walking. Whenever this occurs, take note of where your mind is focused at that moment, and kindly direct the attention back to the act of walking. It may be useful to use the sensation of your feet on the ground, or the relaxed straightness of your spine as a focal point to draw your attention back to the physical sensations that emerge moment by moment. The pace of your walk should now be moderately slow, but reasonably comfortable. In time you may find yourself walking at a more 'normal' pace. Note any tendency to speed up excessively as you would notice any distraction in your mindfulness practice, and gradually allow yourself to return your attention to the physical sensations of walking, anchoring your awareness through your inhale and exhale and with your physical contact with the ground. This exercise can take place over a fifteen- to twenty-minute span. When you have concluded this practice, allow yourself to exhale fully and completely let go of the exercise, giving yourself credit for having engaged in this work, moving towards developing greater mindfulness and compassion.[10]

After working with this exercise for a few days or weeks, you might choose to bring this quality of awareness to other activities, making the transition to applied mindful awareness. In this way we might have the experience of connecting with our observing self as we go through our everyday life.

Challenges on the Path to Mindfulness and Compassion

As you engage in mindfulness training, you will probably come into contact with some obstacles and challenges. This is a normal part of every human endeavour, isn't it? I doubt anyone ever set out to learn to play the violin or the guitar without hitting the wrong notes or having sore fingers. Learning involves stumbling and confusion. A compassionate and mindful awareness of our step-by-step learning can allow us to embrace the process, rather than to descend into self-criticism and shame. As we've discovered, the learning involved in cultivating a compassionate mind involves a gradual development of our inborn, intuitive wisdom and requires patience and consistency. We are not asked to punish or judge ourselves; quite the opposite, really – our work involves a growing acceptance of who we are, fully, in the present moment, as we move towards the cultivation of self-compassion.

So, mindfulness training will pose different challenges and potential problems for each person. Let's take a look at some of these challenges together, so that they might not take us by surprise. Although we might 'intellectually' grasp the notion of non-judgemental awareness, we may still cling to our stubborn judgements. This is to be expected, and is a part of the ongoing process. Remember, mindfulness is the non-judgemental observation of the contents of consciousness, and compassion as a non-judgemental awareness of the observer herself. The challenges we face in cultivating mindfulness and compassion are often things that we can't 'work around', but that we can 'work through'. For example, we might wonder if we have completed a mindfulness exercise 'right' or if we've done it 'wrong'; however, for our purposes, as long as we have allowed ourselves time to sit with our experience, and observe the flow of our attention, we have done the exercise 'right'. Mindfulness is a practice of being rather than doing, and it really is one of the few human activities that allows us to totally let go of the idea of 'getting it right'. I find it helpful, particularly on days when my mind seems too active to sit still, to remind myself of the Buddhist saying that 'as soon as we sit on the meditation cushion we are already enlightened'. Another challenge to practising the exercises is staying awake! For example, the deep relaxation that results from The Body Scan may loll some of my clients to sleep. This response is completely normal but it is important to remind ourselves that, with practice, The Body Scan becomes more an exercise of 'falling awake' than of 'falling asleep'. With practice this will happen naturally, so if you find yourself falling asleep in the beginning, see if you can open your heart with compassionate self-acceptance and just let yourself be where you are in the process. That is much more in tune with our aims than struggling to 'be better'. If you have particular difficulty staying awake during mindfulness work, even after several weeks of practice, you may opt to practise with your eyes open, and direct your attention to a space on the floor or an object in the room that you find comforting. Whatever you need to do to adapt these practices to work for you, the key is that you keep engaging and experimenting and practising.

The aim is for compassionate mind practice to ease your anxiety, and to activate your affiliation system – that accepting soothing system within yourself to form a secure base from which to operate in the world with compassion and courage.

Although mindfulness can be relaxing, people often report that they feel anxious or experience difficult emotions during their daily practice. Sometimes this can make it seem as if the mindfulness-training techniques 'didn't work'; but, in fact, bringing mindful awareness into contact with anxiety may be exactly *how* this practice works. During the practice of mindfulness the aim is to fully experience whatever may unfold before our minds, moment by moment, in a spirit of willingness, curiosity and openness. This is different from pushing away and avoiding uncomfortable experiences or from attempting to control our emotions. By experiencing our anxiety in this new way, we are opening the door to compassionate attention, and preparing ourselves to come into greater acceptance of who we are and rest in the presence of our compassionate minds. We may actively learn that attempts to control and suppress anxious emotional experiences may actually be amplifying and perpetuating our distress. Mindful acceptance and compassionate attention directed towards ourselves can help us to break this cycle and help us cope with our experiences.

In traditional Buddhist writing on mindfulness and liberation from anxious suffering, we can find five potential roadblocks to cultivating mindfulness. These obstacles are sometimes known as the 'Five Hindrances'.[11] Let's take a look at each, try to find ways to work with these natural human tendencies and open the door for compassion.

The first of these hindrances involves a craving for pleasurable experiences. The pull of something appealing in our environment or even in our imagination can persistently draw us to be hooked by the craving for and fixation with desirable or exciting thoughts, images and experiences. This natural tendency can distract us during mindfulness training but when we notice these distractions and preoccupations, we simply need to make space for them, acknowledge them, and bring our attention back to the present moment with our next inhalation. We may need to repeat this several times, but each time knowing that we are practising a new way of relating to an experience that can dominate of our thoughts, images and feelings and, as a result, our behaviour. We are also practising the ability to observe and balance our emotion-regulation systems, allowing for the eventual activation of our compassionate, affiliation system.

The second of these classical Buddhist hindrances is 'ill will', which refers to our preoccupation with memories of painful emotions, our emotional and physical pain (or discomfort) in the present moment, and our concern about pain in the future. This can be anything from a persistent itch or cramp to a nagging memory of a lost opportunity. Our habitual entanglement with our painful experiences, irritants, coldness or itching, and anything generally unpleasant to us can be a persistent and challenging distraction but we can meet these distractions by using our mindful acceptance and, after exhaling, return to the present moment.

In these first two hindrances, we can see how our attachment to having what we want and getting rid of what we do not want both conspire to redirect and distract us from our engagement with the present moment. Through the development of mindfulness and compassionate attention, we can work with these two hindrances by anticipating the pull of sensory experiences, by recognizing that this is a natural part of being human, and that it is not our fault. Reflecting upon our practice, we can recognize that both pleasant and unpleasant inner experiences might arise during mindfulness training, and that both can be met with flexible, focused, non-judgemental attention, and by again and again returning our attention to the simple, open observation of each individual moment.

The third hindrance to meditation practice is anxiety and restlessness. We can see, in this hindrance, the activation of our threat-detection system, and the ways our 'always on, better-safe-than-sorry' problem-solving machine can get a hold of our whole being, narrow our attention, and shift us away from the directions of our valued aims. While practising mindfulness, the threat-detection system can result in the fidgeting that emerges when we try to keep our bodies still. Mindfulness training gives us the opportunity to notice and to take action to change these habitual patterns. Through mindfulness, we can practise staying in the presence of anxious agitation, remain open and aware and bring compassionate attention to our experience throughout the process. This is the first step in our conscious activation of our compassionate emotion-regulation system.

The fourth hindrance is known as 'sloth' or 'torpor' and represents low energy levels, a state of exhaustion, and a general slowness to respond. This hindrance may manifest itself as 'lazy' avoidance, as procrastination, or as the symptoms of low energy and exhaustion that can so often accompany depression or the feeling of being overworked. When we encounter this during our mindfulness practice, we might simply be tired or possibly have overeaten. However, this experience may also be the result of a strong aversion to fully experiencing some unprocessed emotions that might show up during the practice. Scheduling and commitment to practise even in the face of an urge to procrastinate can be very helpful in overcoming this problem. Working with a teacher, therapist or sharing these experiences with others who are practising mindfulness training can help us work through these problems. In my own experience, I often have felt 'too tired' to practise mindfulness, or 'haven't had the energy' to sit. When I hold myself, gently, to the commitment that I have made, and practise mindfulness for even a few minutes, I often find that I have much more energy, and a much greater sense of ease, after sitting. There is no guarantee this will always be the case, but I do find it an encouraging experience, and it helps me return to my practice when my mind is telling me to just avoid it.

The fifth and final hindrance is described as 'doubt' or 'indecision', which means that it is challenging for us to commit and have clarity of purpose in our practice. When we aren't sure of the outcomes, we often go back and forth over what to do. Indeed, we humans aren't comfortable with ambiguity. We've evolved to treat something that *might* be bad as if it *were* bad. Part of this might be related to a discomfort with uncertainty, which is characteristic of people with chronic worry known as Generalized

Anxiety Disorder. This doubt may also involve self-doubt, arising from a negative belief about one's own abilities and strengths. In this, we can see the activation of the blaming and shaming parts of our threat-detection system. Part of the aim of our mindfulness training involves our gradual acknowledgment of such doubts as part of the flowing landscape of the mind. So our work lies in applying mindful awareness to whatever arises in this moment. In this way, we won't need to surrender control of our behaviour to the stream of emerging private events that continuously presents itself in the mind. This will result in a flow of compassionate attention that forms the foundation for our work in developing the compassionate mind.

Having used mindfulness training as the platform for the development of compassionate attention, we can now move on to further compassionate mind-training exercises: cultivating our capacity for compassionate imagery, compassionate thinking and compassionate behaviour.

7 Compassion-Focused Imagery

When we are faced with the intensity of our anxiety response, we often crave relief and escape. Unlike dangers from the outside world, fighting or fleeing from our anxiety, worry and panic can amplify and deepen the activation of our threat-detection system. If we are wracked with anxious suffering but if escape and avoidance makes things worse, where are we to go, and what are we to do?

So far, we have begun to explore other ways of addressing our threatened minds. Our work has led us to a point where we can directly train our minds to activate the capacity for compassion, calm and courageous acceptance steeped in warmth and inner strength. We are beginning to learn how to direct this capacity to the experience of anxiety. This takes time, and means that you will be working directly with your experience of anxiety. This process can sound intimidating, yet we are bringing a very powerful ally along with us on this journey: our compassionate, tolerant minds.

The skills and attributes of the compassionate mind can help you focus on the present with a sense of strength and stillness, even when things seem to fall apart around you. Your compassionate mind stimulates a part of yourself that possesses courage and authority when faced with fearful situations. When we use our compassionate minds we are awakening an evolved capacity to operate effectively while still in the presence of our anxiety. One of the most powerful tools that we have in cultivating the compassionate mind is our capacity for imagery, which can be used to help us activate different emotions and physical sensations. For example, we have seen that what we focus our attention on can affect how we feel. When our minds begin to imagine things our whole being can respond as though this mental event had actually happened and this often gets us into trouble with anxiety. We might imagine a potential disaster, become fearful, and then avoid the situation we worry about. If we are hungry and imagine a meal, we can stimulate our salivary glands. Similarly, if we imagine scenes of a sexual nature then we may feel aroused. This basic human ability for our imagination to stimulate systems in our brains and bodies can also be harnessed to stimulate our compassionate minds and, in turn, our soothing system. And, crucially, if we engage with compassionate imagery then we can activate systems in our brain that will help us tolerate and cope with anxiety.

Many of my clients say, 'I can't do imagery; I'm no good at it.' The simple act of guiding our imagination can seem too difficult and, as we know by now, it doesn't take long for us to start judging ourselves if we find something difficult. Nevertheless, I've found that resistance to the use of imagery to build self-compassion is usually driven by people misunderstanding what imagery actually is. Often, people think they have to create 3-D, HD pictures in their minds or cinema-sized screens in their heads! As if some special talent and excellence were called for. But this is not what we are after. Imagery, basically, is fleeting, impressionistic and unique to each person and it's the emotions and the focus of our attention that is really important during exercises that use our imagination. If I ask you what your car looks like, what image would pop into your mind? If I asked you what you had for breakfast how clear and perfect an image of your cereal bowl would arrive? If I asked you what kind of summer vacation you would like, how would you reply? Any answer uses imagery, which appears in your mind. It might not be sharp and may only be fleeting and fragmentary but that's all you need. The clarity of the image is not important; rather, it is the sensations and feelings that emerge that we are interested in.

Imagery, or visualization, has been used for millennia by different cultures: ancient Hindu priests would visualize the fire within them and feel the warmth of a divine presence; Jewish mystics visualize the presence of God in themselves and in the universe; within the Christian tradition there are many examples of prayers that evoke and involve visualization; in Buddhist contemplative practices there is a long tradition of using specific visualizations to access parts of ourselves, such as our compassionate self, in order to alleviate our suffering. Similarly, CFT uses visualization to help activate and engage our compassionate selves and our affiliative emotion-regulation system so that it is ready to deal with and cope with what matters most to us in our lives. CFT techniques, however, are drawn from evidence-based psychotherapy methods, the neuroscience of emotions, behavioural theory, and evolutionary science, rather than solely on ancient cultural traditions. This allows us to test and explore the hypotheses that have guided and driven spiritual and philosophical practices for centuries, and to continue to discover how best to alleviate and come to terms with our struggle with anxiety.

The following series of exercises can be used as an introduction to compassionate imagery, but can also be adopted as regular, daily practices in training our compassionate mind. Many of the same principles of structured, consistent practice that we have learned in the previous chapter will be helpful but for now I would suggest that you take the time to experience each of these exercises for yourself. If you are working with a therapist or teacher you might want to discuss your responses to the imagery with them. If you are working on your own, you can document your observations. Recordings of these exercises can be found at www.mindfulcompassion.com. It is important that you begin to practise these exercises at a pace that feels comfortable. As you become familiar with one series of exercises, feel free to move on to the next series.

Exercise: Creating a Safe Place

This first compassionate-imagery exercise, 'Creating a Safe Place', has two functions. First, it helps direct our attention towards the sense of feeling safe. The practice of imagining a safe place for ourselves allows us to explore and be curious about what kind of things will be important to us to evoke feelings of safety. Sometimes, if we're feeling a bit stressed out, taking time to just imagine a safe place can give us somewhere to rest. Secondly, creating a safe place helps us imagine somewhere that gives us a sense of joy. For example, because this place is your creation and is from your own imagination, it is a place that welcomes you, possibly – as one of my clients described it – as if it's a place where your dog wags its tale and barks happily to welcome you when you return home. But you need to find your own ways of thinking about it. The place you create is meant to embody compassionate warmth and safety. In this exercise, we are allowing ourselves to experience feelings of being safe already, of already abiding in place where we are relaxed and confident about our well-being.

When we feel anxious, a sense of contentment and security may seem miles away; however, our minds respond to our imagination as though what unfolds may be real. We have learned that we have evolved to feel comfort in the presence of strong supportive attachment figures who can activate this sense of safety, and we know that in this way we have an inborn capacity to use our imagination and cultivate feelings of safety and activate our self-soothing system.

Instructions

It is a good idea to begin this exercise as you might begin the soothing-rhythm breathing, by lying comfortably on a mat or sitting in a comfortable, secure posture on a chair or meditation cushion. Take some time to allow a few mindful breaths to move in and out of the body. Now, turn your attention to your imagination and begin to think about a happy, secure place that surrounds you. Perhaps it is a place you have visited, somewhere from your past, or even somewhere you have only thought about visiting. It is important that this place represents somewhere calm, such as in a shady picnic spot, or a seaside balcony, or a cosy chair by the fireside in winter; whatever it may be, this place is just for you, and you are free to imagine anywhere that feels right to you.

If you imagine a serene sandy beach, feel the smooth, soft sand beneath your feet and the warmth of the sunlight. Do you hear the waves lapping against the shoreline? Or the seagulls calling?

If you imagine somewhere secure, cosy and warm indoors, such as a comfortable chair beside the fire, can you feel the heat radiating out to warm you? What does it smell like? Can you hear the fire crackling?

You may remember somewhere you have walked among ancient trees and greenery, or somewhere else that holds fond memories for you, when you were supported, loved and able to experience a sense of playfulness. In order to vividly evoke such images, recall what it was like, or what it may be like if you were actually there, right now. Notice the quality of the light, the texture of the sand, the fabric of the chair, the bark of the tree, and notice the sounds, smells and temperature.

Remain with this visualization for a few minutes, and from time to time note the natural rhythm of your breathing, feeling your diaphragm and belly rising and falling with the even pace of the breath. Whenever your mind wanders, draw your attention back to the image of your safe space with the next natural inhale. After a few minutes, allow the image to fade, and gradually let go of the entire exercise with the next natural exhale, and return your awareness to your actual surroundings.[1]

Exercise: The Compassionate Self

This next exercise will help you imagine yourself in a very different way than you might be accustomed to, as if you are an actor who is rehearsing a role in a play or a film. The exercise involves the creation of the personification of your compassionate self, who you will meet and who will be happy to see you.

Building and becoming the compassionate self

Let's take a moment to think about the qualities our compassionate self by writing down the qualities you would ideally like to have if you were calm, confident and compassionate. Would you be wise? Strong – and able to tolerate discomfort? Would you have warm feelings towards others, and towards yourself? Would you feel empathy for someone else's suffering, and for their behaviour? Are you understanding of others faults and foibles and as a result non-judgemental, accepting, kind, forgiving? Do you have courage? Ask yourself how you would picture your most compassionate aspect. Perhaps you might imagine yourself older and wiser, or younger and more innocent. This is *your* exercise, and you are free to embellish and design an image of your compassionate self according to your own desire.

To begin, find a place where you will feel safe and may remain uninterrupted for some time. Ideally, this would be a quiet and special place, such as the one you might use for your mindfulness practice. Start the exercise as you would your soothing-rhythm breathing. Allow your eyes to close; bring part of your attention to the soles of your feet as they connect with the floor and to your sit-bones on the chair. Allow your back to be straight and to feel supported. Next, partly direct your attention to the flow of your breath in and out of your body; allow it to find its own rhythm and pace. Feel yourself breathe in, and breathe out. Continue this breathing uninterrupted until you've gathered your attention and feel focused on the present moment.

At this point, recall the qualities of your compassionate self that you wrote down, and now *imagine that you already have* those qualities. Breathe in as you experience yourself making a wise decision; breathe out. Breathe in and imagine yourself courageously confronting your fears; breathe out. Continue through the list and then imagine all these qualities together, and your ability to be compassionate towards yourself, and towards others. Imagine yourself as a completely non-judgemental person who doesn't condemn yourself or others for their faults or foibles. Allow yourself to bring to mind the sensory details that you would notice as your compassionate self. What are you wearing? Is your body relaxed and receptive? With body language that signals openness and kindness? Are you smiling? If not, smile now, and at the same time imagine the warmth you feel when you carefully hold an infant. As you breathe in, bring attention into your body, imagine yourself expanding, and welcome your ability to be wise, warm and resilient.

For the next few moments, as you are breathing in and out, imagine what the tone of your voice would be if you were this compassionate self. How would you behave? What would the expression on your face be? Allow yourself to take pleasure in your capacity to share kindness with, and care for those around you, and yourself. If your mind wanders, as it so often does for all of us, use your next natural inhale to gently bring the attention back to this image of your compassionate self.

Our aim in this moment is to connect this image you have created with the compassionate image of you at your very best. Can you see the two people standing side by side, and then merging into one? For the next several minutes continue to give mindful attention, returning and refocusing when needed, to this compassionate self. When you feel ready, and with your next natural exhale, allow any attachment to this exercise to simply melt away. Breathe in again, and with the next natural exhale allow yourself to become aware again of your surroundings and then recognize and acknowledge the effort you have invested in this exercise. As you let go, fully return your attention to your surroundings and carry on with your day.

I'd like to take a moment to put our work here in a little bit of historical context. In Buddhist art there are paintings known as *mandala*, which display the Buddha and other mythological beings within a series of circles. These mandala represent a map of the inner world of a human being and are symbolic of the various aspects of our personalities: of our wisdom, our rage, our joy, and even our lust.

A mandala or other such images can be used as part of a special meditation that employs visualization, sound, and certain small gestures to help evoke the various parts of ourselves so that we may come to terms with all aspects of our being, and from a broader perspective. The idea is that if we focus our thoughts (in terms of mental images), words (mental or verbal phrases with special meanings) and deeds in the form of unique gestures that connect us with a particular experience, we can then later recall certain aspects of our personality that may help us deal with times when we are suffering.

Bringing the Compassionate Self into Contact with the Many Parts of You

There are many different parts of who we are: our angry self, our anxious self, our joyful self. Let's begin our soothing-rhythm breathing and then pause for a moment to reflect on this.

In order to understand the various parts of personalities, and the way they affect our behaviour, it may be helpful to separate these various aspects and look at them individually. For example, imagine having an argument with somebody who you know to be harsh and critical. What does the angry side of your personality think about this situation? How does it feel in your body to feel criticized or attacked? What behavioural urges arrive in this angry part of yourself? And if this angry part of your personality seized control of things, what would it do?

Now, bring your attention back to the flow of your breath and with your next natural exhale let go of this image of the angry self.

With your next natural inhale, focus on your anxious self and how it might deal with the same argument. What does the anxious part of you think? What are your physical sensations? What would this anxious part of your personality do if it seized control of your behaviour?

Now, bring your attention back to the flow of your breath and with your next natural exhale let go of this image of the anxious self.

With your next natural inhale, let's focus on the interaction between your angry self and your anxious self. Do they like one another? Does your angry self approve of what your anxious self and how it behaves? What does your anxious self think about your angry self? Is it frightened of it? Does the anxious part feel protected by your angry self? And does the angry part feel threatened or stifled by the anxious self?

Now, bring your attention back to the flow of your breath and, again, with your next natural exhale let go of this image of these two parts of your personality.

All these different parts are really just the way we deal with events as they unfold. Often, these different parts can be in conflict with one another, and make us feel in conflict with ourselves; however, when we activate and connect with our compassionate self, things can be quite different. At this point, rather than focusing on the anxious or angry aspect of your personality, let's focus on the wise, calm, authoritative and compassionate part. Pause and rest in the flow of your breath, and spend a few moments focusing on this part of you. See yourself from the outside with a gentle smile on your face, and see other people relating to you as someone who is calm, kind and wise. Once you have got the sense of this aspect of yourself, imagine this compassionate self dealing with that initial argument. What are your thoughts about the argument now? How does that calm, wise and compassionate self feel? What is this compassionate self doing when it takes control of your behaviour? How would this be different to the way your angry or anxious self behaves?

Now, bring your attention back to the flow of your breath, exhale and let go of this image.

When different emotions flow through us they affect the way we feel about ourselves by affecting our thoughts, physical sensations and our behaviour. We can let them do their own thing of course, and let our anger or anxiety run the show – it might seem easier to hand over control; but in the long run it's not so helpful or compassionate towards ourselves to do so. Compassion gives us courage to take control and hand back our behaviour to the parts of us that we know will help us to lead our lives calmly and with kindness towards ourselves.

This exercise might have given you a glimpse of what happens when you start to deliberately and willingly focus your attention towards the kind of self that is likely to be helpful to you.

The chances are that if you suffer from high levels of anxiety, you're very familiar with your anxious self and possibly also your angry self. You may be familiar with how you become angry with yourself for being anxious and anxious when you become angry, and less familiar with the way your compassionate self deals with the problem of anxious suffering. But this is what these exercises and practices will help you do: discover how your compassionate self deals with, or helps you cope with your anxiety.

By this point we have done a lot of work to develop an understanding of the nature of anxiety. We have learned where it comes from and how it can take control of our thoughts and behaviours and that it is *not your fault*; that your 'always on, better-safe-than-sorry' threat-detection system is ready to leap in and take control partly because of the way our brains have evolved and partly because of our personal histories. These tricky complicated brains of ours do allow us to negotiate our way in the world but we are better off when we understand them somewhat. Thankfully, we also have a capacity for cultivating our self-compassion and our mindful attention to our compassionate selves. By learning how to do so, by embodying and manifesting the strength and wisdom of our compassion, new things become possible, and our outlook broader.

Exercise: Experiencing Compassion Flowing In

Find a place to begin this next exercise where you can sit with your back straight and supported, either in a comfortable chair or on a meditation cushion. Much like our other exercises in mindfulness and compassion, it is good to find a quiet space, where you will be undisturbed for about ten to twenty minutes, when you can allow yourself to devote some attention and energy to yourself.

Start by bringing attention to your breathing by observing its flow and rhythm and allow the breath to find its own pace. Observe and remain with this flow for a few minutes.

Next, bring part of your attention into your body, and feel the strength and compassion that is available to you in your posture. Feel your feet on the floor, your sit-bones connected to your cushion or chair, and your spine straight and supported. Your posture is grounded, dignified, and reflects your sense of calm and self-compassion. Allow your face to form a gentle smile and with part of the attention staying with the flow of the breath begin to remember a pleasant day in your past when someone was compassionate and supportive towards you. This person was non-judgemental, didn't condemn you, was empathic, and cared about you and your happiness. As much as you can, remember the sensory details of this experience. Can you remember what you were wearing? Where were you? Was it hot? Or cold? Or raining? Was the wind blowing through the trees or the radio on in the background?

Now, bring your attention back to the flow of your breath, inhale and exhale and stay with this image for a while.

We are now focusing our attention on our desire to be kind and help-ful and we do this by remembering the experience of receiving such help and kindness. Whenever your mind is inevitably distracted, and wanders away from this memory, gather your attention with the next natural inhale, make space for whatever is arising, and simply return your attention to the breath and to the image of this compassionate person with your next natural exhale. As you breathe in again, with your next natural inhale, bring your attention to the facial expression of this person from your past. Allow yourself to remember, as much as you can, their body language and movements. What did this person say to you? How did they say it? Pay particular attention to the tone and sound of their voice. Stay with this experience for a little while, breathing in and out. Next, bring your attention to the quality of the emotion this person had for you. How did they feel towards you? How does this make you feel – do you have any physical sensations as a result of your emotion? Take a few minutes to remain in the presence of that emotion. You may feel safe and protected, or feel as if your body is grounded and stronger. However this emotion shows up, see if you can welcome it, identify it as mindful compassion, and invite yourself to make space for it. This is a time to bring attention to the experience of compassion flowing into you.

Now, bring your attention back to the flow of your breath, inhale and exhale smoothly and take a few moments to stay with the way this experience feels.

As much as you can, connect with the emotions of appreciation, gratitude and happiness that arrived with this person's care. For as long as feels right to you, perhaps a few minutes more, remain in the presence of this memory and this feeling. When it feels right, let this experience go and with your next natural exhale allow the memory and images to fade away. After a few more slow and even breaths, exhale and let go of this entire exercise.

Before you open your eyes and resume your day, take a moment to give yourself credit for engaging with your practice of self-compassion, recognizing that you have made a conscious decision to take care of yourself, and move towards the alleviation of your suffering from anxiety.

Exercise: Compassion Flowing Out

This exercise will allow you to build upon your practice of mindful, compassionate attention, and develop your experience of using imagery to activate your affiliative self-compassionate system. As we begin, we will engage in the same practices that form the first stages of our soothing-rhythm breathing. Finding a quiet and safe place, we adopt a dignified, meditative posture, with the soles of our feet connected to the floor, our sit-bones on our chair or cushion, our back straight and supported. Start by following the breath in and out of the body and become aware of your physical presence, just as it is, in this very moment. Allow the breath to find its own rhythm and pace. Whenever our attention wanders, we can gently and consistently draw our attention back to this moment, by focusing again on the breath.

After a few minutes, as you have gathered and collected your attention in a mindful and compassionate way, bring your attention to a time when you felt compassionate towards another person when they were in need of a helping hand. You can even bring your attention instead towards the compassion you felt for an animal, for example a pet. Remember this as a time of relative peace and happiness. Although we often direct compassion towards our loved ones during times of distress, this exercise involves using imagery to evoke a feeling that is separate from difficult emotions. As you imagine feeling kindness and compassion towards others, see if you can imagine yourself expanding as the warmth and care of your intention grows. Imagine that you are becoming a wiser, emotionally stronger and warmer person with each inhale and exhale. As you become more mature and resilient with every breath, recognize that this means with each breath you have more to give, that with each moment you are becoming more helpful, open and wise. How does this feel? What physical sensations are you having?

Now, bring your attention back to the flow of your breath, and focus on these feelings and this image for a moment longer, all the while observing your desire for this person to be happy, for them to be filled with compassion, for them to be peaceful and at ease, and for them to be well.

What is your tone of voice like? What is the expression on your face? How is your body moving and reacting to your feelings and to the feelings of the other person? Take some time to enjoy the sense of pleasure you may feel by being helpful and caring. Remember to smile gently and as you breathe in and out, allow yourself to notice the sensation of compassion flowing out of you so that it reaches this person whom you care so deeply about. Imagine your compassion touching their heart. Imagine the burden of their suffering is lifted little by little with every breath. With your next natural exhale, sense again the compassion flowing out of you, and joy and peace flowing into the person who you are sharing kindness with. With your next natural exhale, let go of this representation of the other person and draw your attention simply to the experience of compassion in yourself. Recognize where in the body your open and heartfelt desire to share kindness and helpfulness presents itself. Allow yourself to rest in this feeling of loving kindness for others, feeling the presence of compassion for others as it flows through you. Stay with this sensation for a few moments more.

If your attention wanders at any point simply pay mindful attention to where it has gone but then refocus by bringing part of your attention to your next natural inhale and to the exercise at hand.

After some time, when you have remained in the presence of this warmth and kindness for a number of minutes, you can return your awareness to your feet on the floor, your position in the chair, to your back, straight and supported, and ultimately to the top of your head. When you feel you are ready, exhale and let go of this exercise, giving yourself some credit for having engaged in this practice. You may wish to jot down some of your observations in your practice diary or journal. If you are working with at therapist, meditation teacher, or other people who are practising compassionate mind training you may wish to share some of your observations and experiences with them.

Exercise: Creating and Encountering the Compassionate Ideal

Many people who struggle with anxiety have had troubling emotional experiences involving their caregivers; others will struggle with anxiety-related emotions that relate to their negative experience of affiliation. This in turn leads to fearful and destructive behaviour and difficulty with creating a compassionate self. Such a fear of self-compassion and a lack of experience of kindness can be a powerful and poignant obstacle to the activation of our capacity to regulate our emotions.

As a result, CFT practitioners understand that it is best to learn compassion in small steps, gradually building a capacity to evoke self-compassion, and to activate positive, calming emotions when faced with elevated levels of anxiety. So, we have begun with exercises that involve relatively small steps, which can be seen as a sort of hierarchy of exposure to compassion itself; after our initial training in mindfulness, we began to explore mindfulness training by using visualization, when we imagined a safe place we could return to in our minds when we are feeling distressed or anxious. The next step involved the construction of our image of a compassionate self whose qualities include such things as empathy, tolerance to distress, wisdom, patience, and the ability to be calm and to show kindness. By focusing on our compassionate selves we are getting in touch with our affiliative soothing system, and training ourselves to access this system when we need it – at any time or place. Following the construction and awakening of a compassionate self, we learned how compassion towards the self may be evoked by using our imagination and memories to experience compassion flowing into us, as well as to experience compassion flowing out. In these practices, the use of imagination was directly connected to our emotional experiences and activated our emotion-regulation system.

Our final exercise involves creating an image of a compassionate ideal who you can relate to through visualization and who becomes an inner helping hand and shoulder to lean on during times when you are distressed and anxious.

Start by practising your soothing-rhythm breathing. Take a few minutes to bring mindful, self-compassionate awareness to the flow of your breath. In this moment, allow your awareness to follow the natural, calming rhythm of the breath as it helps you focus on the present moment.

Drop your tongue from the roof of your mouth, relax, and feel the muscles of your face form a gentle smile. As you have in your other exercises, allow your posture to feel grounded to the earth, supported, and embodying the qualities of dignity and supple stability.

You may wish to think about your compassionate, safe place where you can feel yourself surrounded by a sense of emotional warmth and where you can begin to form the image of your compassionate ideal.

The image of your compassionate ideal is built up, gradually, from elements of your imagination and experience. The image can be very personal, and it is meant to have significance to you and for you alone. If your compassionate ideal changes over the course of this exercise, fine. You may even develop more than one image. For now, though, settling into the present moment, let's draw our attention to the qualities that you would like to see in this particularly compassionate ideal.

Begin by asking yourself what qualities really make you feel cared for, protected and soothed. And remember, this is an ideal image that we are breathing life into; we don't need to be concerned about how realistic our expectations are. This ideal is our own, personal, mythical being, closest friend, superhero or guardian angel. Sometimes people use the image of the ideal parent but keep in mind this image will never criticize you or be angry with you. We are creating a compassionate ideal based on the qualities we would wish to encounter in the experience of mindful compassion flowing into us.

Some qualities you might wish for in your compassionate ideal include a deep reservoir of inner strength and the ability to tolerate and contain anxiety and distress without being overwhelmed and with immovable compassion and calm, even in the presence of great pain and fear.

Your compassionate ideal will embody a deep commitment to alleviate your anxiety and pain and takes pleasure and satisfaction when you experience joy and happiness. The greatest desire of your compassionate ideal is to help calm your suffering and anxiety, and to bring you peace, warmth and contentment.

Your compassionate ideal represents and personifies wisdom and understands that life is very hard, and that none of us chooses to struggle with anxiety, an emotion common to everyone. Emotional pain and fear is our common bond, and you can sense that this compassionate ideal has learned through experience that suffering is not our fault. After all, we didn't choose to be here, nor did we choose to evolve with such very complicated brains, filled with strong and confusing emotions and motivations. We didn't choose our personal histories or our painful memories. Knowing all of this, your compassionate ideal truly understands the complexity of the life you face and is filled with abundant kindness and a broad, accepting perspective.

When you are in the presence of this compassionate ideal, you can sense the great warmth that this image embodies. You can feel patience, understanding, caring and kindness emanating from the presence of this image. Your compassionate ideal is also absolutely accepting of you, exactly as you are, here and now. This compassionate presence never condemns you, never judges you, and holds you in perfect and unwavering kindness, now and forever, without condition or reservation.

As your mind encounters each of these qualities, allow them and the sense of them to wash over you as you follow your breath in and out of your body.

As you continue to form the visual image of your compassionate ideal, ask yourself if this guiding presence is in the form of a human being or if it is in the form of a mythical creature or animal. Perhaps your compassionate image represents aspects nature, such as a radiant pure light, or the ocean. How old is this image? Is it youthful and innocent? Older and wise? Or ageless? Is it male or female? Or neither? What might this image be wearing? Would they be dressed or adorned with colours or textures that feel soothing? Add to this image as much as you desire and allow yourself to connect with your compassionate ideal's ultimate and absolute intention, which is to be completely committed to the alleviation of your suffering. Your compassionate ideal wants nothing in this world so much as for you to find happiness, live in peace, and experience well-being and joyfulness, in this moment.

As you allow this image to form in your mind, rest in the soothing flow of your breath and take a moment to let your imagination simply be in the company of this compassionate ideal, who is directing all their kindness and attentions towards you. As your breath follows its rhythm, allow your mind to repeat the following words, which come from your compassionate ideal:

May you be filled with compassion and kindness; may you be well; may you be peaceful and at ease; may you be free from suffering; may you be happy.

Imagine these words flowing from your compassionate ideal into you with each inhale and then, with each exhale, release any tension or struggle within yourself. Simply let go. Stay with this image of your compassionate ideal and this recitation, and this flow of the breath, remaining in the calming presence of your compassionate ideal for as long as feels right to you.

When you are ready, and with your next natural exhale, gradually allow this image to fade, and return your attention to the soothing rhythm of your breath. When the time is right, give yourself some credit for having engaged with this practice of creating a compassionate ideal, and let go of this exercise altogether with your next natural exhale.

Using Compassionate Imagery in Everyday Life

As we have seen, there are several exercises that help us find and use compassionate imagery. In these meditative-like practices, we begin with a gentle focus on the rhythm of our breath, and use our imagination to activate our soothing, compassion-focused emotion-regulation system. This kind of gradual practice can develop our ability to calmly, compassionately and courageously face our anxiety, worry and fear; however, we aren't limited to working with compassionate imagery purely through formal exercises. For example, once you have begun to have a clear and accessible image of your compassionate self or your compassionate ideal, you may find it helpful to pause for a few moments when you are feeling distressed or anxious, and bring one of these images to mind. You might then imagine yourself having a soothing and encouraging conversation with your compassionate self, feeling the emotional tone of warmth and helpfulness that this part of yourself brings into your mind and heart. Responding in this way will allow you to build a new range of responses to anxiety over time. This also lays the foundation for compassionate thinking, and the range of thought-based techniques that we use in CFT.

8 Compassionate Thinking

Moving from the Anxious Mind towards Compassionate Thinking

As we explored together in the first half of this book, anxiety involves the activation of our threat-detection system, and involves attention, physical sensations, thoughts and emotions. Our thoughts can become extremely negative and provoke even more fear and dread when we are anxious. These thoughts can stir up a common form of anxiety-driven thinking typically referred to as 'worry', which involves generating representations of things that could go wrong in the future, and which usually takes a 'what if' format: 'What if I lose my job?' or 'What if I get cancer?' or 'What if I can't make any friends?' As we discussed, the ability to generate a range of possible threats in our imaginations, and to prepare a number of protection responses has much to do with how we've evolved to face and deal with threats. When our hypothetical risks and dangers show up, we often take the projections of our minds literally but when these worries arrive they can stir up or compound distressing emotions, and control our behaviour. Our attention narrows to focus on these thoughts, and we may then have a narrower range of possible behaviours available to us. So, yes, this kind of thinking may have its evolutionary usefulness, but it isn't often very helpful for us now.

Compassionate thinking brings our compassionate self to the aid of our anxious self by helping us see things, or think about things, in a different way. Our anxious self might be quick to jump to conclusions, because of its orientation to be 'better safe than sorry'. It will also be bound to our memories; so if we've had a bad experience in the past the anxious self will remind us about that and reactivate those feelings of fear and dread; however, when our compassionate attention alerts us to the onset of anxiety, we can choose to move towards compassionate thinking to help us face our worry, fear and panic.

Let's take a closer look at this process to see how we can actually work with compassionate thinking to take care of ourselves when we respond to anxiety.

Imagine that you are stuck in heavy traffic, which is causing you to run late for an important meeting. Suddenly you start to feel panicked; your stomach tightens and maybe you have a tingling in your fingers. At the same time, your anxiety generates thoughts such as:

- Oh my god, I'm starting to feel bad; I might be sick.

- What happens if I have to throw up and I have to lean out of the car?

- I'm stuck in a traffic jam and I can't pull over!

- This is terrible, unbearable. What are they going to think of me at the meeting? I've been trying to set up this deal for weeks and now this happens! What if it falls through?

- Oh no, my heart, it's racing. What if I'm having a heart attack and die?

Actually, just writing this makes me feel a bit of anxiety in my chest. We know it's scary when even the words evoke some fear in us. But what would you do, how would you react and feel if you engaged your compassionate self right now?

Firstly, let's focus on practising soothing-rhythm breathing, which will help our breath slow down. Just for a moment, let's find a place to rest in the breath. When we get anxious we tend to speed up our breathing and it becomes shallow because of the tension in our body. This can also evoke some of the symptoms in the body of feeling anxious, such as tingling of the skin, nausea and light-headedness. We aren't attempting to banish our anxiety or struggle against it in an effort for control. We are simply preparing the way for our compassionate self and coming into the moment with a warm-hearted acceptance, as much as we can.

Next, take on the posture of dignity, and create a friendly facial expression, even if you don't really feel like it. Imagine being in the safe place where you have been practising your exercises. Does that help? Imagine your compassionate self in the safe place and then moving from that safe place to where you are now, in this moment. This is the compassionate self who is going to help you as you face this situation. Now think about how you would love to be able to respond to this anxiety. How would you understand, tolerate it and get through it? Sure, who wouldn't want to 'get rid of it' and magically make the traffic start moving again, but *unfortunately* that doesn't usually work, particularly in the long term. It is far better to learn how to tolerate anxiety, ride it like a wave, and recognize that we don't need to be scared of it even though it is frightening. For the moment, imagine yourself coping as the ideal, compassionate self. What would this compassionate and wise self be thinking? Would it be calm, and try to help you also to be calm? Try some of these thoughts and see what you think:

- I have felt anxiety like this before, many times, and I know that I can feel claustrophobic – I recognize these feelings as my threat-detection system doing what it has evolved to do. It is unpleasant for me, but is a part of life. (*Always remember to validate what you feel. Recognize the suffering.*)

- These anxiety feelings are not my fault – they are partly related to the way my brain is built – and also to things that have happened to me in the past. Maybe I am experiencing panic now because my life is very stressful at the moment so my anxiety threshold is weakened. (*This is helping you understand the context and nature of panic.*)

- Many people suffer panic attacks – not just me. (*This is learning to constantly remind yourself that as much as you hate panicking you suffer from it along with many millions of other people. You are not alone.*)

- I have had these feelings many times before and they do pass and subside – I can bring to mind times when I have panicked in the past and when it's then gone away. Let me just hold that memory of successfully coping in mind. (*This is helping you learn to see your panic as part of life's journey and that it comes and goes.*)

- When people are panicked it's very common for them to believe something terrible is going to happen as a result but, in fact, panicking doesn't kill you. Our bodies are designed to cope with feelings of panic. There is no evidence that people who've suffered from panic attacks are more at risk of dying from heart attacks than other people. (*This is helping you hold on to the evidence about the difference between feelings of panic and having heart attacks.*)

So you see the key process here involves validating your feelings while being kind to yourself and recognizing them as unpleasant. You don't need to tell yourself that you are being silly or neurotic or pathetic or that you just have to grin and bear it, because thoughts like these are not very kind or supportive, are they? Also, while it understandable that we get irritated and angry with our anxiety ('Why does this have to happen now? What the hell is the matter with me? I hate feeling like this!'), your task in evoking your compassionate self is to be at your *most supportive*.

Sometimes, though, learning not to panic can be helpful, and one way to do this is to connect with your sense of wisdom, authority and a real commitment to try to be helpful, not on trying to come up with the most accurate assessment of the situation. Imagine yourself as if you were hovering slightly above the anxiety and then expanding to capture the anxiety. Can you see how much bigger you are than the anxiety? When you do, you will be able to watch your experience of panic unfold in safety.

Sometimes it can be useful to imagine how we would help a friend who was in a state of panic; however, if you're unsure of how to help yourself it can be difficult to know what to say to a friend. But if you learn how to be kind to yourself, and to support yourself with acceptance, you can become understanding, kind and supportive to others also.

So run through these thoughts in your mind, but always keep those feelings of deep understanding, courage, kindness and warmth because your compassionate self knows how scary panic is. Your compassionate self will not be dismissive of how you're feeling or what you're thinking.

Here's an experiment – read through the alternative thoughts set out above, as if you were testing them out for whether you believe or not? Rate them on a scale of 0–10, with 0 being not helpful at all and 10 being very helpful.

Now, close your eyes and engage your soothing-rhythm breathing, a soft facial expression, and imagine talking with a friend in a firm but kind tone of voice. Sit upright in the chair with your back straight and supported, and engage with your sense of dignity and strength. Next spend a moment or two imagining seeing your compassionate self from the outside. See how you stand, how you talk, how you look and how people relate to you. Then bring yourself back into being this compassionate self, with as much warmth and kindness as you can. Next, refocus on those alternative thoughts very slowly indeed, and on the genuine desire to be helpful with the difficult feelings you are experiencing – don't rush it, and continue to breathe rhythmically and calmly.

What did you notice? Did you find yourself feeling more grounded and more able to tolerate anxiety when you used your compassionate self to help you? Remember, too, that every time you make this compassionate and courageous effort to cope with your frightening thoughts you are strengthening your connection to your compassionate self.

Exercise: Bringing Compassionate Thinking Closer into Contact with Worries and Anxious Thoughts

When we use the word 'worry', we are referring to the way our anxious mind will generate predictions about what might go wrong in the future. Our threat-detection system cooks up worries in the form of 'what if' sentences that can provoke a great deal more anxiety and fear in us. See if any of these 'what ifs?' sound familiar to you from your own experience of worried thinking:

- What if I never find a job?

- What if nobody wants to date me, or be with me?

- What if I get sick?

- What if I lose my pension savings?

Of course, our anxious mind is very good at generating anxiety-provoking predictions of possible threats. All too often, our emotional brains then respond to these imaginary threats as if they were real, so our physical sensations, feelings and behaviour come to be dominated by our worries. Let's take a look at how compassionate thinking can help us address our worries and anxious thoughts in clear and useful ways.

First, it helps if we consider what our anxious mind is actually focused on and explore our thoughts from flexible perspectives. To do this, we can ask ourselves a series of questions. In traditional Cognitive Therapy this is sometimes called 'guided discovery'. Here are some examples: 'What is going through my mind when I am anxious?'; 'How does my anxious self see the world, and what does it think about the current situation?'; 'What is my anxious self most anxious about, right now?'

As you begin to practice this kind of questioning, it is sometimes useful to write these thoughts down and then imagine your compassionate self, with its wisdom, sense of authority, calmness and genuine desire to care. How would your compassionate self respond to these thoughts? How would the presence of self-compassion guide your discovery?

For example, let's imagine that you have to give a presentation to your colleagues. The prospect of this stirs up your anxiety, and your mind begins to generate worry and fantasies of the presentation going horribly wrong. You ask yourself, 'What if I just freeze?', 'What if I really screw this up and wind up getting fired?' You might hear your mind saying such things, but because you are so close to the experience it seems as if these thoughts present real threats and may come true, instead of being *events in the mind*; however, you are learning now to give yourself a chance to step back by asking yourself, 'What is my mind telling me right now?' After all, we don't need to believe everything that we think! We can, instead, bring our thoughts before the witness of our compassionate self, and shift our perspective.

It can be helpful to write down your thoughts and generate alternative thoughts in response to stress and anxiety. This can help you develop the skill of compassionate thinking. There is a worksheet at the back of this book called 'The Compassionate-Thought Record' which may help you record your distressing thoughts, and to come up with new ways of responding to them. The rest of this chapter, including a practical exercise, will help you learn a range of techniques to move towards compassionate thinking using the Thought Record as a bit of a road map. It's important to remember, though, that when we are aiming to think differently in compassionate mind training, we aren't looking to just dispute our thoughts, test their validity, or to become 'more rational'; the aim is to develop a self-compassionate, mindful experience of warmth, self-acceptance and kindness.

Techniques for Engaging Compassionate Thinking

As you might expect, compassionate thinking is interwoven with many other compassionate attributes and skills. It necessarily involves building on our training in compassionate attention and compassionate imagery. Let's take a look at an example of how compassionate thinking can be applied to an anxiety-provoking situation. Imagine that my client Jennifer is going for an interview for a new position as a history teacher at a different school. She has a stable job, but this new one would be a big step-up and an exciting new opportunity. So, despite her apprehension about interview situations, Jennifer has decided to take a chance and apply for the position. She arrives early for the interview, and sits in the waiting room for a few minutes before the appointed time. She begins to notice that she is feeling apprehensive, nervous and fidgety. Her mind is beginning to race with worries and predictions of failure; however, Jennifer has been practising her compassionate-thinking exercises and begins to respond to these feelings by taking a few mindful, soothing-rhythm breaths. She allows herself to rest in the breath, and asks herself: 'What is my anxious self/mind telling me right now?' Stepping back from the flow of her anxious thoughts, Jennifer is able notice that she is having the fearful thought that: 'I'm going to mess up this interview and it's going to be a total disaster!' But because she has gathered herself into the calm flow of soothing-rhythm breathing she is better able to recognize this thought as on that is associated with her feelings of anxiety and her threat-detection system, rather than as a fact. After all, she has prepared for the interview, and she has the experience and credentials that would make her suitable for the position.

With part of her attention still focused on the gentle rhythm of her breath, she next imagines herself *as* her compassionate self and asks herself what this wise, kind and helpful aspect of herself might say in this situation. Beyond this, she might also have a sense of what it would feel like, emotionally, to be in the presence of this compassionate friend. Sitting in the waiting area, Jennifer imagines that her compassionate self tells her: 'Jennifer, it is completely natural that you would have some feelings of anxiety or fear in this situation. Job interviews can be anxiety provoking for all of us. We have evolved with such complex minds, and our anxiety can be activated so quickly, so this is not your fault, and you are OK just the way you are. Remember that you have prepared for a long time, and that you are competent, caring and knowledgeable. When we think about it, you actually do have a job already, and you are doing very well there. As much as you can, just make space for the ups and downs of what you feel, and hold yourself in kindness and care, just as I do.' After imagining these words, Jennifer recalls the sensations she has experienced during the Compassion Flowing-In exercise, and connects with a sense of mindful self-compassion. She recognizes that by stepping out of her comfort zone to come to this job interview she has begun to engage in compassionate behaviour. She is being kind to herself, courageous, and putting up with feeling anxious in order to move in a new and meaningful direction.

Developing the skill of compassionate thinking takes some practice, and that practice can take place throughout the day, as a natural part of your daily life. Sometimes this practice can take place in structured way, through the use of the Compassionate-Thought Record. At other times, you might simply use your creativity and wisdom, without the use of the Thought Record and without writing anything down. Part of our aim in compassionate mind training is to internalize and learn these compassionate-thinking skills, and build your compassionate attributes, so that your new, more helpful response to anxiety becomes automatically and inherently more mindful and self-compassionate.

Let's take a look at three approaches to developing compassionate thinking which eventually will become a part of our broader range of responses to anxiety. These approaches share some common ideas, and also have some distinctions, and they all share the common aim of helping you to activate and embody your capacity for self-acceptance, kindness, warmth, and a deep sense of safety and contentment in the present moment. These three approaches are: Compassionate Responding; Examining the Costs and Benefits of Compassionate Thoughts; and Compassionate Defusion.

Compassionate Responding

In CFT the purpose of alternative responses to anxiety is to notice the flow of anxious and negative thoughts as they move through your consciousness and then come up with alternative, more positive thoughts that adopt a more compassionate perspective, allowing balance, self-care, and movement towards compassionate behaviour. We aim to ask ourselves questions, and shift our perspective in ways that evoke the emotional tone of our compassionate selves, and connect us with our sense of a sense of warmth, wisdom and inner resilience.

You may find it helpful to write down some of your observations as you practise these exercises, and notice how the alternative responses affect your feelings.

Exercise: Compassionate Double Standard

When you notice that you have become anxious, or are feeling distressed, you may begin by asking yourself, 'What is going through my mind right now?' See if you can stand back from the flow of your thinking, and capture the thoughts that are going through your mind in a sentence or two. For example, if you were stuck in traffic and as a result are running late for work, you might feel stress and pressure building up. This is a good time to take a moment to stand back and ask yourself compassionately what you are thinking in that moment. You might notice that you were worrying, and that the 'what ifs' began to pop up: 'What if I'm late? If I'm going to be late, then this is going to be a total disaster. I'm going to be in huge trouble. I've screwed everything up!' The next step in this compassionate double-standard exercise would be to ask yourself an important question: 'What would I say to a good friend who was faced with this same situation?'

As the name of this exercise implies, we often apply harsher rules and standards to ourselves than we would to others. Our inner critic and threat-detection system can be activated by stress, and that can result in reacting to our threatening, worrisome thoughts in less helpful ways than if we were engaging with our compassionate selves. This additional pressure can ramp up our experience of shame and anxiety. By looking at our situation and our automatic thinking as if it were happening to a friend, we can adopt a more helpful, compassionate and kind attitude to ourselves. We can view the situation through the lens of our compassionate mind, and respond with balance, patience and support. If your best friend rang you while they were stuck in traffic and panicked about running late, you might respond by saying, 'That kind of situation can be so frustrating. As much as you can, remember that the traffic is not your fault and is out of your control. You're probably one of hundreds of people stuck on the same route. If you can, let yourself off the hook on this, and just ring your office to let them know you're stuck.' In speaking kindly and supportively to your friend in this situation, you would be helping them both validate their distress as well as move beyond their anxiety and find the best solution to the problem. More than this, you would be providing the support and calming influence that arrives with the activation of our experience of compassion from others, through our contentment and soothing emotion-regulation system. The compassionate double-standard exercise aims to help us be just that kind of supportive friend to ourselves, responding to anxious thoughts and worries with compassion, support and care.

Exercise: Examining the Costs and Benefits of Buying into a Thought, from a Place of Compassion

Like all the techniques involved in building our capacity for compassionate thinking, examining the costs and benefits of buying into a thought begins with the simple act of noticing where our minds are, and what they are doing, in this moment. When we are in distress, or if we notice the physical sensations or emotions involved in anxiety, we ask ourselves, 'What is going through my mind right now?' After noticing the thought, we could write it down at the top of a sheet of paper, and begin to ask ourselves what are the advantages and disadvantages of buying into this thought. We might draw a vertical line in the centre of the paper, and write 'costs' at the top of one half, and 'benefits' at the top of the other half. There is a form provided for you at the end of this section that will help you put this into practice. You can do this in your mind, too, but it may be easier at first to write it out. After reviewing the costs and benefits of believing this thought, you might ask yourself, 'Do the costs of buying into this thought outweigh the benefits? Does it help me to buy into this thought? If I did believe this, how would I behave? Do I want to hand my behaviour, and my life, over to this kind of thinking?' You might consider how your compassionate self would advise you in this.

Taking a few soothing-rhythm breaths, activating compassionate attention, and bringing your compassionate self to mind, you might ask that kind and helpful part of you if believing this thought will serve your valued aims and will lead you to self-compassionate behaviour. If you decide that it is more costly than beneficial to believe in or act upon this thought you can bring acceptance and compassion to your experience of the present moment, see the thought for what it truly is – an event in the mind – and refocus your mindful attention on a compassionate alternative thought that will help you behave in a compassionate, effective and kind way.

Exercise: The Compassionate View from the Balcony

This is adapted from an exercise from cognitive therapy that encourages us to adopt a new perspective upon our thoughts and feelings, by re-imagining the situation we are in. It can be used any time that you notice anxiety or distress building, whether it be in a particular place or situation or completely out of the blue. Sometimes we begin to notice our emotions because of physical sensations such as tension or nausea; at other times because of negative thoughts that begin to swirl around. However you notice your emotions, it is important to allow yourself this moment of observation and ask yourself a central question that helps you engage with and acknowledge your thoughts, such as: 'What is going through my mind right now?'; 'What is my mind telling me?'; 'What am I thinking in this moment?' As much as you can, see if you can catch the thoughts as they unfold in your inner monologue, and observe them as sentences that you can jot down or repeat. For example, after an argument with a friend, you might nervously wait for them to ring and either apologise or talk things through. Or you might be trying to build up the courage to make the call yourself. Feeling the tension in your chest and pressure in your temples, you might notice that you are feeling anxious and angry. Making space for these emotions, you could choose to ask yourself, 'What is my mind telling me right now?' Casting a lens upon your thoughts, you might notice statements such as, 'She's driving me crazy!' or 'I've ruined everything!'

Once you have noticed the things that your anxious mind is saying, you can begin to use your imagination and perspective to work with your distressing thoughts. And this is where the Compassionate View from the Balcony can help you. Imagine that you are at a beautiful theatre, and that you are watching a play from one of the balconies. At one point during the play the lead character is acting out a moment of distress. You have been watching the play for some time now, and you have developed empathy, compassion, and warm feelings for this character. Imagine now though that the character you are watching is actually you. That what you are seeing is a play about exactly the same situation you find yourself in right now. Rather than watching the events and thinking the thoughts from the inside, though, you are now able to have some distance and observe how the lead character has struggled, as all humans do, and that the hero of this play has felt some serious anxiety.

You recognize that this is not the character's fault, that they didn't choose to be in this situation or ask for their anxious suffering, and they never asked to face the difficulties and challenges they are presented with at this point in time. This character has struggled and suffered, and you feel great empathy for them. You understand their pain, and are moved to help them alleviate their suffering. If you were watching these events and hearing these thoughts from this perspective, from this compassionate view from the balcony, how might you respond to the negative, anxiety-based thinking that you sometimes notice within you?

Exercise: The Compassionate-Thought Record

The following worksheet is structured to help you practise compassion-ate thinking every day with questions that can guide you through the steps of compassionate thinking. Of course there will be some times when you can complete this exercise in 'real time', responding to anx-iety and other emotions as they happen by writing down your responses. At other times, you won't have that opportunity, and can complete the worksheet later, looking back on an event from earlier in your day and then rehearsing how you might respond when a similar event happens, or reflecting on how you were able to use compassionate thinking to help you cope with your anxiety during the situation. With practice, this written format will help you shift from anxious to compassionate perspectives as an automatic response. Feel free to experiment with this exercise, and to share your observations with your therapist, if you are working with one, or with people you trust who are helping you on your journey. Alternatively, you may wish to keep some of these observations private, and just for you.

It is important to remember that all the skills and attributes of our compassionate mind are connected and that your work with mindful attention and compassionate imagery has established a foundation for your work with compassionate thinking.

The Compassionate-Thought Record
Questions to ask yourself:
1. **What is the situation I find myself in?** In this moment, here and now, what situation do I find myself in? What am I doing? Where am I? Am I interacting with anyone? What do I see, hear, feel and notice around me? What am I reacting to right now?
2. **What physical sensations am I experiencing?** Turning my attention inward, what physical sensations am I experiencing right now? Allowing myself to make space for these experiences, mindfully engaging in the soothing-rhythm breathing practice, can I allow myself to experience these sensations with kindness? What sensations might I associate with anxiety or other emotions?

3. **What emotions am I feeling?**
   If I observe these sensations, how would I label the emotion I am feeling now? What words would I use for my current emotions? How intensely am I feeling these emotions on a scale of 0–100?

4. **What is my mind telling me?**
   What is going through my mind right now? What thoughts are popping into my head? What is my mind telling me?

5. **Can I mindfully and compassionately make space for this experience, here and now?**
   Continuing to engage in soothing-rhythm breathing, and bringing to mind an attitude of warmth and self-acceptance, I am taking this opportunity to learn to stay with my experience, just as it is. Following the flow of my breath in this moment, as much as I can, I am making space for whatever unfolds before my mind. I know that I am more than my thoughts, emotions, and bodily sensations, and that I can let myself recognize that I am a part of the flow of life, and that this is not my fault. I can recall how my compassionate self feels, and hold myself in acceptance and kindness, right here and right now. In the space below, I can write down any observations I make as I do this.

6. **How might I respond through compassionate thinking?**
   How might I best respond to my thoughts and emotions in
   this moment, with compassion, wisdom and acceptance? Am
   I being non-judgemental? What might help me come closer
   to compassionate thinking? What reactions and observations
   have I noticed from the perspective of compassionate
   thinking?

7. After engaging in compassionate thinking while feeling
   anxious and distressed, what do I notice about my current
   emotions, thoughts, body sensations and behavioural urges?
   What is happening for me, right now?

Distinguishing Self-Criticism from Compassionate Self-Correction

For many of us, self-criticism is large part of our inner life. Our learning histories may have involved experiences that taught us to believe negative messages about ourselves, and cause us to feel shameful or not worthy. Such experiences might include being a child of abusive parents or being bullied, or other forms of physical or sexual abuse. Perhaps we have experienced neglect or abandonment. When our caregivers treat us with contempt, cruelty or violence, we might then react to the experience of a relationship with an activation of our threat-detection system. If we look for compassion and safety from others but are instead punished or mistreated, this can lead to us learning to block or fear the experience of compassion and affiliation. This can also lead to an over-activation of our threat-detection system, and a pervasive experience of shame and self-loathing and an active inner critic.

It seems that we are designed to blame ourselves when we have difficulty dealing with our fears and with our perception of threats, which can feel overwhelming. Our problem-solving minds try to find some source of control, some method of finding certainty in the midst of anxiety and danger, and we often blame ourselves if we are not able to find that source or are not able to take control. We have evolved to draw upon whatever resources are at hand to make ourselves safer.

Remember that through compassionate mind training we are aiming to shift the centre of gravity of our experience from threat-detection emotion-regulation towards the activation of our compassion-based system. As our emotions, thoughts and behaviours are interwoven, when we operate from a place of compassion, our thinking takes on a different character and emotional tone, as does our behaviour.

We did not choose our evolutionary history, nor did we choose the learning history that has led us to struggle with anxiety and shame. Developing the compassionate mind begins in the present moment, with the recognition that the situation we find ourselves in is simply not our fault, and with a choice to accept ourselves fully, just as we are, without any condemnation or judgement and compassion for our struggles. When I've introduced this idea to many of my clients, they have resisted it strongly. They believed that by accepting themselves fully, and realizing that their anxiety and suffering is not their fault, they would no longer care about how they treated themselves or others. For some, the idea of compassionate self-acceptance seems to involve self-indulgence, selfishness or a lack of responsibility. In fact, these qualities are not at all part of how our compassionate mind functions. Research has demonstrated that people who have a high degree of self-compassion are actually less self-indulgent than others.[1] Operating from our compassionate minds means that we have a deep appreciation of the suffering of both others and ourselves. We recognize our common humanity, and are moved to do something to alleviate this suffering. This involves consciously taking responsibility for our actions, and plotting a course of compassionate behaviour for ourselves that can live up to the heartfelt aspirations that emerge from our compassionate selves.

Many of my clients also believed that they needed to be harshly self-critical if they were going to better themselves, that if they bullied or beat themselves up, they might whip themselves into shape, and become more motivated to take charge of their lives. This is a common belief. Perhaps you have memories of teachers or coaches who tried to motivate you through derision or harsh criticism. It may have seemed to work but in fact this kind of verbal punishment rarely produces a positive behaviour change. Such punishment often results in a decreased frequency of positive behaviour, not an increase of it. More often than not, our attacks on ourselves, in the guise of 'whipping ourselves into shape', actually have the effect of narrowing our range of behaviours and increasing our anxiety, rather than helping us live our lives more calmly, evenly and effectively. If we allow ourselves to be engulfed by our anxious thoughts and feelings, and if we surrender our behaviour to our fear or to avoidance, we are not actually living from a compassionate intention; however, if on the contrary we train our minds to respond with compassionate thinking, adopting compassionate self-correction rather than verbally attacking or criticizing ourselves, we will be better able to respond to our experience of anxiety and shame. Training our compassionate mind can help us experience positive emotions more readily, overcome anxiety, and more effectively pursue our goals.

The table below outlines some of the differences between self-criticism and compassionate self-correction.

Compassionate Self-Correction is Focused on	Judgemental Self-Criticism is Focused on
• The desire to improve • Growth and enhancement • Looking forward • Generosity, encouragement, support and kindness • Building on positives (e.g. seeing what you've done well and considering what you've learned from other things that would benefit from improvement) • Positive attributes and specific qualities of the self • Hope for success • Possibilities for increasing the chances of engaging with the compassionate mind Note the example of an encouraging supportive teacher with a child who is struggling (below).	• The desire to condemn and punish • Punishing past errors and often looking backward • Meanness, anger, frustration, contempt and disappointment • Deficits and fear of exposure • Fear of failure • Possibilities of avoidance and withdrawal Note the example of a critical teacher with a child who is struggling (below).

From *The Compassionate Mind*, Gilbert, 2009; reprinted with permission.

Compassionate self-correction is grounded in the desire to alleviate suffering, and to help us realize our heart's deepest desire to be able to behave as we would wish to. Paul Gilbert has illustrated this difference by contrasting the style of two imaginary teachers who are working with young children. The first teacher believes that it is beneficial to focus on the deficits and faults that a child might have and that teasing and chiding her pupils for their mistakes will help them learn. Her students come to fear and resent her when she looks over their shoulders at their work, and she herself spends a lot of time feeling angry and anxious about how her students are performing. In contrast is the second teacher, who pays a lot of attention to the strengths and talents that her students demonstrate. Her expectations are clear, and she gives specific behavioural feedback to the children about how they could improve their performance. She does not chide them or tease them. She is encouraging, warm, strong and wise. Did you have teachers like this when you were at school? Which one did you study harder for? Which one did you prefer? Which teacher might have shaped your sense of self-confidence, and as a result help build your capacity to respond to frustration and anxiety with warmth and ability to tolerate distress?

Compassionate self-correction is not about denying our mistakes or our weaknesses; instead, it focuses on radical self-acceptance of our fallibility, our frailty and our suffering, all of which are essential aspects of our common humanity. Such acceptance also involves a deep kindness and appreciation of our desire to alleviate our suffering, to grow, to develop and to realize our valued aims. 'Compassionate self-correction is based on being open-hearted and honest about our mistakes with a genuine wish to improve and learn from them. No one wakes up in the morning and thinks to themselves, "Oh, I think I will make a real cock-up of things today, just for the hell of it." Most of us would like to do well, most of us would like to avoid mistakes, most of us would like to avoid being out of control with our temper. We need to recognize that our genuine wish is to improve.'[2]

The following exercises represent a few methods for overcoming self-criticism through developing our capacity for compassionate self-correction. You can experiment with them as part of your compassionate mind training practice and record them in your practice diary. Like all of the techniques here, feel free to approach them gently and with a spirit of curiosity. Part of the way we cultivate our capacity for compassion is to gradually build new ways of responding to anxiety, and doing so at a pace that works for us. Along this path, we are discovering which techniques speak to us and help us move towards greater acceptance, mindfulness and flexibility. It is a good idea to record some observations in your practice diary about your responses to the different exercises, so that you might be able to follow a course of personal growth and healing that feels right for you.

Exercise: Two Chairs for Your Anxious Inner Critic and Compassionate Self

This next exercise involves noticing the different parts of ourselves, particularly our anxious mind and our compassionate mind and then drawing a contrast between the two. We are going to use a form of role play to create a dialogue between these aspects of the self. By doing this, we can feel what it is like when we are spoken to by our anxious self, and then experience how dramatically different this is to speaking with our compassionate selves. In addition, this will help us practise activating our compassion system, which can help us cope with our fear and anxiety.

You will need two chairs, which should be placed facing one another. As you begin, sit in one chair, and imagine that you are looking at a mirror image of yourself in the other chair. Take a moment and connect with your feelings of anxiety and self-critical thoughts and then speak directly to this other image, as if you were the personification of the anxious and self-critical part of yourself. Your words will involve shamefulness, worry and bullying. You might be familiar with this kind of dialogue already, with prior experiences of similar thoughts. When you are ready, speak to the empty chair, all the while continuing to imagine that you are facing yourself and remembering that you are speaking purely from your anxious, self-critical mind, and are giving a voice to your threat-detection system. Speak your fears, your self-criticism and your worries out loud. Let yourself say things that you might not be comfortable saying typically. Feel free to verbalize your anxiety, your shame and your self-criticism as openly as you can. Continue doing this for a few minutes and then, when you are ready, allow yourself to stop speaking. Take a moment and settle into your chair, letting some silence pass after you've spoken.

Next, and again when you are ready, rise up and take a seat in the opposite chair. Close your eyes and allow yourself to settle into a few mindful breaths, resting in your soothing-rhythm breathing. Bring to mind the image of your compassionate self and allow a gentle smile to form on your face. Make sure you are sitting in a grounded and dignified posture, and then call to mind thoughts of acceptance, forgiveness, openness, warmth and kindness. Allow these thoughts to become physical sensations, perhaps with a feeling of warmth around your heart, or your smile broadening. If it is helpful, you can even place your hands over your heart for a few moments as you follow your breath, and hold the image of your compassionate self in your mind. Now, open your eyes and look at the chair before you and begin to speak completely from your mindfulness and compassion, and acknowledge that you are speaking with your anxious self. You are not chiding or bullying or criticizing; instead, you acknowledge and accept the fear of your imaginary self sitting opposite you, and you speak with wisdom, emotional strength, kindness, and the ability to tolerate the distress of this anxious self. For example, you might say, 'I understand how difficult this experience is for you. You are very frightened; you aren't sure if this experience will be worthwhile. It is hard, and you are anxious, and I get that. But please remember that it is not your fault. I hold you in kindness, and have a real wish for your happiness and well-being. It is OK for you to feel this way.' Stay with this compassionate voice for a few minutes more and then, when it feels right, close your eyes and with your next natural exhale let go of the exercise altogether. When you open your eyes, bring your attention back into the room and allow yourself some credit for courageously engaging with this practice.

This exercise can seem a bit strange or tricky at first, but with a little practice you can begin to learn what it is like to deliberately activate your compassionate mind, and to respond with compassion and self-correction when you experience fear, anxiety and self-criticism arising within you. With regular practice, compassionate self-correction becomes something automatic in you. Your range of possible responses to self-criticism can broaden, and you can find a new freedom to bring self-compassion into the present moment as you face your anxiety and self-criticism from a place of safety, strength and wisdom.

Exercise: Writing a Compassionate Letter to Yourself

This exercise will involve writing a letter to yourself from the perspective of a deeply compassionate, wise, and unconditionally accepting person. If you feel comfortable, you can imagine yourself as this loving, kind presence. This voice within you is an expression of your innate loving kindness and intuitive wisdom.

In preparation, set aside some time when you can engage in this exercise without interruption and without hurry. Find a space that feels private and safe and where you have a surface to write upon. You could use some of your good stationery and one of your good pens, or simply use a pencil and a clean sheet of paper.

As you begin, take a minute or two to engage in mindful awareness of the flow of the breath. Sit so that you can feel the soles of your feet touching the ground and where your back is straight and supported and where, overall, you are comfortable. Focus on your soothing-rhythm breathing, paying attention to the movement of your breath in and out of the body.

After a few minutes of mindful breathing, shift your attention to the flow of your thoughts and as you breathe reflect on your current life situation. What conflicts, problems, or self-criticisms come to mind? What is your mind beginning to tell you? What emotions arise within you?

With your next natural exhale let go of these thoughts, and on the next natural inhale shift your attention again to an image of yourself as a compassionate and wise person who possesses wisdom and emotional strength. You are unconditionally accepting of all that you are, in this moment, and are completely non-judgemental. Your compassionate self radiates emotional warmth. For a moment, recognize the calmness and wisdom that you possess and the physical sensations that accompany this. Recognize the strength and healing quality of a vast and deep kindness. Recognize that this loving kindness, this powerful compassion, exists within you as an abundant reservoir of strength.

Remember to acknowledge and validate your feelings and remind yourself that there are many good reasons for the distress you are currently experiencing. Your automatic pilot has evolved to make you feel and react as you do. You were not designed to deal with the particular pressures and complexities of your current social environment. Your learning history has presented you with strong challenges, and situations that have caused you pain. Can you open yourself to a compassionate understanding that your struggle is a natural part of life, and that it is not your fault?

Reflect on this and then, when you are ready, allow yourself to compose a letter that gives a voice to your compassionate self and which will fill at least one page of A4-sized paper, or both sides at least of your special stationery. If you are working with a therapist, you may choose to take this letter with you to your next session, when you can read it together and reflect upon the words and feelings that you have allowed yourself to express. If you are working independently, set aside some time to mindfully read this letter back to yourself with great care. Let yourself hear the words and feel the emotional tone of compassion. If you feel the need to write drafts of this letter several times, please feel free to do so. And please remember that each time you are practising one of your CFT exercises, you are learning to come into closer contact with your compassionate emotion-regulation system, and are gradually developing your compassionate mind. So, feel free to practise as often as you wish, and as often as you can.

Compassionate Defusion

Defusion represents our ability to break away from what we have learned in our past to be our mental content, and begin to live by following our valued aims and by engaging in mindful and compassionate attention, thinking and behaviour. We are removing and breaking – 'de' – with what we have been connected to – 'fused' with. When we practise compassionate defusion we are taking the time to rest in our soothing-rhythm breathing, to come into contact with our compassionate self, and to adopt a new perspective about the way we think. With self-kindness, recognition of our common humanity and a willingness and capacity to bear distress, we can experience our thoughts as events unfolding in our minds, rather than something our anxious self must hand our lives over to.

As we have discovered, when we think about or imagine something, our bodies and minds can respond as though the mental image were a real thing in the outside world. For example, if you imagine that your favourite food has been set down on the table before you, with the wonderful aroma of a fine freshly prepared meal, you might salivate or notice that you are getting hungry. Similarly, if you tell yourself that 'I am a going to embarrass myself at this party' or 'I can't get on that airplane' you might feel anxious or afraid. And as our bodies begin to feel the physical effects of anxious thoughts, we then begin to feel even more distressed. Our threat-detection emotion-regulation systems become the captains of our souls, and we become immersed with the experience as if it were a literal event; however, because of the various mindfulness training exercises we have been practising, we have begun to be aware of how helpful it can be to simply not take our thoughts at face value; to stand back and imagine ourselves as compassionate and wise; and to bring in kindness to balance our thoughts. By doing this, we will begin also to defuse ourselves from the way our thoughts present themselves, and reclaim control of our behaviour from the domination of thinking that is led by our threat-detection system.

Practising compassionate defusion allows us to use our mindful, compassionate attention to gain perspective of the thoughts and emotions that flow through us, to separate ourselves from these thoughts and consider how they are affecting us. We may benefit from becoming ever more observant of our inner experiences for what they are and not for what they try to convince us they are.

You'll find below a number of defusion techniques that can help you to practise broadening your range of responses to anxious thinking.

Exercise: Breaking from Identification with Thinking

Your foot is a part of you, but it isn't all of you. When you have a dream, that dream unfolds in your mind, but it isn't 'you'. Similarly, our thinking and verbal minds are a part of who we are, but they aren't all of who we are. For this exercise, imagine that your mind is something outside of yourself, almost separate from who you are; for example, you might think, 'My mind is telling me that I need to stay inside today' or 'Oh, my mind is doing its old familiar pattern of worrying about my retirement.' It can also be helpful to talk through your emotional responses by saying out loud or to yourself: 'My mind is telling me that I'm going to fail this test, and that's generating a flash of anxiety. This means that my body has picked up a perceived threat. I can see how this is working to make me feel butterflies in the stomach. Let's see if I can just make space for this experience for a moment. I can notice how these thoughts are pulling my feelings around but I'm going to return my focus to studying, as much as I can, and as often as I need. I can contain all of this right here and now.' By learning to stand back from your experiences, with non-judgemental observation, you are gradually learning to defuse from the flow of mental events, rather than over-identify with them and hand your life over to anxiety. Call to mind a physical sense of warmth and the strength and wisdom that emerges from self-kindness. Understand that you are not merely the thoughts that float across your mind. You are something much bigger, much more important, and something that can contain this experience. Holding yourself in kindness, practise this defusion with the flow of your thoughts, and explore what happens.

Exercise: Taking Your Keys with You

This next technique involves linking your mental events to an object in the outside world. Grab your key ring and match each anxiety-provoking thought and feeling to one of the keys: your house key represents worries about your relationship; your car key might represent worries about your finances; your office key might represent worries about your health. It really doesn't matter which key goes with what; what matters is to link each thought with one of the keys, and experience the thought in a new context. As you go about your day, recognize that you are carrying these sometimes troubling mental events with you just as you are carrying your keys. You need to carry your keys in order to function in your day, just like you need to carry these thoughts. Notice the thoughts, and your ability to carry them, whenever you notice the keys. When you notice your mind returning to these familiar worries, bring part of your attention to the keys and feel them. Remember that with mindfulness, compassion and acceptance, you can carry these thoughts just as you carry the keys, using them when you need to and putting them away when you don't in order to open and close doors that lead you in different directions throughout your life. Connect with your sense of compassionate tolerance of distress as you do this, recognizing that your compassionate self has sufficient warmth, wisdom and strength to hold your anxious experience, help you move towards what matters most to you, and away from what doesn't.

Exercise: The Children on the Bus

Let's begin this exercise by imagining that you are a bus driver. You have your uniform, your shiny dashboard, your comfortable seat and a powerful bus at your command. This bus represents your life: all of your experiences, your challenges and strengths have brought you to this role. You will be driving this bus to a destination of your own choosing – a destination that represents the valued aims that you are willing to pursue. Arriving at your destination is deeply significant to you and every inch that you travel towards this valued aim means that you have been taking your life in the right direction. As you are driving, it is necessary that you keep to your course and follow the correct path. Like any bus driver, you are obliged to stop along the way to pick up passengers; however, the trouble with this particular journey is that some of these passengers are difficult to deal with – they are the most unruly and aggressive children you have ever encountered. Each one represents a difficult, anxiety-provoking thought or feeling that you have had to contend with over the course of your life. Some of the children might be self-critical; others are panic and dread; still others represent worry and fear. Whatever has troubled you and distracted you from the rich possibilities of life is now hopping on your bus in the form of these unruly children, who because of their behaviour seem cruel and rude: they shout insults at you and throw rubbish all over the place. You can hear them calling: 'You're a loser!'; 'Why don't you just give up? It's hopeless; we'll never get there!' One even shouts, 'Stop the bus, this will never work!' You think about stopping the bus to scold and discipline these children or throw them out, but if you did that you would no longer be moving in the direction that matters to you. Maybe if you made a left turn and tried a different route the children would become quiet. But, this too is a detour from living your life in a way that takes you towards realizing your freely chosen, valued aims. All of a sudden you realize that while you have been preoccupied with devising strategies and arguments for dealing with the nagging children on the bus, you have already missed a couple of turns and have lost some time. You now understand that in order to get to where you want to go, and in order to continue moving in the direction that you have chosen in life, you need to continue driving and allow these children to continue their catcalls, teasing and nagging all the while. You can make the choice to take your life in the right direction, while just making space for all of the noise that the children generate because you can't kick them off, and you can't make them stop.

You recognize that each child represents a part of your very tricky brain that has evolved over millions of years to respond in all sorts of anxious, angry and confusing ways to a complicated environment and you decide to take a moment to pay attention to the road and rest in the rhythm of your breathing. When you do this you can recognize that it isn't your fault that these painful thoughts, emotions and experiences show up. Your compassionate self, driving the bus, can make room for them all: the anxious self, the angry self, the cruel self, the jealous self, and the entire range of different aspects of your experience, all of them carrying on and vying for your attention like so many restless and mischievous children. All of this can take place as you move towards your valued aims. Importantly, you are being kind to yourself and non-judgemental as you keep your eyes on the road.[3]

9 Compassionate Behaviour

By now we have learned that compassionate behaviour involves a deep awareness of the presence of suffering in ourselves and in others, coupled with an ever-emerging aspiration to alleviate that suffering. We have looked at compassion as an aspect of our minds that has evolved to provide us with a secure base to face the challenges in life, and to move towards what is truly important for us and for our loved ones. We have also learned that our compassionate minds can help us regulate our emotions and cope with our anxiety. We have also seen that compassionate mind training involves working with our attention, imagery, thinking and behaviour as well as our emotions and motivation.

What really moves us along in overcoming anxiety is learning to behave in new ways in relation to it. We used the example previously of learning how to drive a car, when you knew that the only way you would improve and overcome your anxiety would be to get in the car and practise how to drive. Remember also the other things in your life that have happened as a result of your ability to face up to your anxiety (such as taking exams, going for your first job interview or first date). You got through them all and achieved things you wanted, or at least made an effort to; however, compassionate behaviour is not just what you do but how you do it. So, for example, if you suffer from agoraphobia, part of you will want to go out and overcome your fear but another part of you will want to avoid those situations where you might feel anxiety and panic in the outside world. Compassionate behaviour is about choosing to go out, even if it's difficult. Why? Because it helps you stop suffering by being trapped in your home. You might develop a programme where day by day you try to get out, perhaps first by going to the door to look down the road and then tomorrow by taking a few steps to the pavement or to the post box.

The more you create an understanding voice in your mind that validates and recognizes how unpleasant anxiety is, and helps you keep in mind all those things you learned about anxiety in the preceding chapters, the more you will be able to stay with the anxiety rather than have the anxiety push you back into the house. You will be better able to remember new responses such as staying in contact with the present moment, paying gentle attention to your body and your breathing, noticing when you jump to frightening conclusions, noticing when you become self-critical, acknowledging what you've noticed and then refocusing on your compassionate, mindful self.

All our behavioural changes are important because they build confidence in us. The key, however, is to be able to develop a behavioural programme for yourself that is challenging but not overwhelming and which allows you to see that it's OK to take two steps forward and maybe occasionally one step back as you learn to cope with your anxiety.

Why Bother? Clarifying Your Goals and Valued Aims

It is clear that when we begin to engage with our anxiety it's going to be uncomfortable for us. So the issue is: why bother? Well, bear in mind that there is no absolute rule that says you *have* to address all your anxieties. Suppose you have a fear of flying but it doesn't matter so much because you prefer to travel by car or train, when you enjoy the journey, or because you prefer not to travel far and have no need to fly, or because plane travel is not something you need to do for work. In this case, you might not see any reason to overcome your fear. Many people carry with them all kinds of fears that they don't particularly want to engage with, because these fears don't really interfere with their lives. So, the first thing for you to do is to clarify your valued aims and goals for working with anxiety and which parts of your anxiety and fears need to be focused on; for example, you might want to reduce your social anxiety because you want to go to university and become involved in campus life. You might want to overcome panic attacks simply because they're so unpleasant. It can be helpful to clarify what you want to achieve, especially when the going gets tough. When things seem difficult on the road to our valued aims we can keep in mind what we are trying to achieve, and why. Otherwise, it's can be easy to lose motivation and a sense of perspective when we become anxious.

As we look closely at ways to cultivate compassionate behaviour in our lives, we discover that identifying our heart's desire about how we truly wish to behave in our world is a big part of activating the compassionate mind. We also learn how compassion can involve courage, discipline and sacrifice as well as joy and warmth to help us experience whatever shows up for us in the present moment, be it anxiety, uncertainty or fear of the unknown. Even in the presence of distress, engaging compassionate behaviour involves perseverance and moving towards what matters most, with an expanding range of behavioural options. Compassionate behaviour towards yourself may take obvious forms such as:

- Taking care of yourself whether by having a relaxing massage or by taking time out to spend time with people you love.

- Taking care of your health by visiting the doctor or by exercising regularly.

- Taking a break from a stressful situation to relax and enjoy other activities that bring you pleasure.

These are the kinds of sensible behaviours that don't really put any pressure on you and which are often quite easy to do; however, facing your anxiety though self-compassionate behaviour can also take less obvious yet very important forms, for example:

- Working hard to move in directions that you value in life, like studying for exams or pursuing a career, even when this is uncomfortable, and involves sacrifice of time or energy.

- Facing up to things that scare you so that you might overcome your anxiety, even though this involves distress.

- Refraining from taking part in 'pleasurable' activities that might harm you, such as drinking a lot of wine at a party to 'take the edge off' or 'calm your nerves' when you know this activity will have negative results in the long run.

Let's take a closer look at some specific examples of compassionate behaviour, and take part in some exercises that are designed to help you activate your compassionate mind and motivation.

Gradually Developing Compassionate Behaviour

Compassionate behaviour involves taking action, and specifically doing those things that will be helpful and supportive for us in the face of anxiety. This kind of behaviour emerges from a compassionate motivation, a genuine desire to alleviate the anxious suffering that we experience in ourselves and others. Compassionate behaviour may involve soothing ourselves and others, but it also may involve moving in the direction of our valued aims, even when this means we will confront our anxiety head-on.

Just as we have seen with the development of the compassionate mind in general, the development of compassionate behaviour often proceeds in a gradual, step-by-step, course. For instance, I remember a time when I decided to practise yoga regularly again after many years of sporadic, or nonexistent, involvement. One of the things that became most clear to me once I began was that I couldn't push myself beyond where I was actually able to go, nor to where I had been able to go when I had practised regularly in the past. I could only stretch and breathe into a position as deeply and as fully as was possible in that moment. It made no sense for me to try to push myself farther than I was capable of and to damage my body. In time though I became much better able to move through the postures and connect with my breath. This led to better energy levels and improvement in my physical health; however, I had to allow the process to happen gradually, gently and with a blend of self-kindness, non-judgement and perseverance that involved the development of a form of compassionate behaviour.

It takes time for us to identify and understand what matters most to us, and to develop the practice of mindfulness and compassionate behaviour that will help us reach our valued aims and goals.

Self-Compassion in Action

By now, we know that we can develop our compassionate mind to help us feel soothed, content and calm. We also know that this involves courage, strength and authority, which in turn provide a secure base from where we can face challenges. It is important to remember that we are not developing our mindful, compassionate selves to allow us to curl up into a ball and hide away. Instead, we are developing a secure base of self-compassion that will allow us to confidently pursue our valued aims and return occasionally to a safe place that will enable us to rest, to survive and to thrive, even when our anxiety begs us to turn back. Our ancestors might have been seeking things from this place such as shelter, food or safety from predators. In contrast, many of us now live in a world of surplus; however, we still are on the hunt of food or other goals, and we still must contend with predators – more to our spiritual selves than to our physical selves.

When I write about 'values', 'valued aims' or 'valued directions' in this book, I am using the term 'value' to represent behaviour that is intrinsically rewarding across time and across situations, as your 'heart's deepest desire for how you want to behave in the world'.[1]

We all have things specific to us that seem to light a fire beneath us and our values reflect the degree to which certain behaviours are reinforcing our values, which in turn relate to the consequences of our actions. Let's take a look at a few examples of how values can influence our interactions with our environment and with anxiety:

- Steve, who has great experience and skill with computer technology, doesn't really care about financial accomplishments. He values helping people achieve their education goals. As a result, he has said no to the offer of a high-pressure, high-paying job that would require long hours and has taken on another position that pays less but which allows him time to volunteer at a local school to tutor underprivileged children.

- Jane highly values her ability to be a good parent but has an intense fear of social situations; however, because of her values she is willing to face her fear and agrees to meet up with the other parents in her neighbourhood so that her children might make more friends and have play dates with other children from their school.

- Jacob is a talented artist and has been accepted on to a sculpting course that will help develop his skills and possibly lead to commissions. He is also afraid of travelling in confined spaces such as the subway; however, this is the only viable route to the studio and because he values both his work and the teaching he is receiving he has been able to confront his fears, even though it has been very difficult, and has meant that he has had to cope with his anxiety by focusing on his aim (the completion of the course) even when he sometimes experiences panic attacks en route.

Research has demonstrated that when people engage more fully in behaviours that give them a sense of pleasure and mastery, they can begin to overcome negative emotions. In fact, these kinds of behaviours may be more effective in overcoming negative emotions than psychiatric medication or than some therapeutic treatments for depression.[2] Research has also indicated that what most effectively changes our negative thinking is engaging in behaviours that help us move in the direction of our valued aims[3] and that by doing so, even in the presence of distress, we can also help ourselves to overcome our problems with anxiety.[4] So, in order to engage in truly compassionate behaviour, and take good care of ourselves, it is very helpful for us to move in the direction of our own valued aims.

Let's take a moment now to discover what valued aims and directions are meaningful and worthwhile to you. What are you willing to experience anxiety and fear in the service of? What behaviours are intrinsically rewarding to you? If you were to be compassionate towards yourself, and courageous in your pursuit of your valued aims, where would you be headed? In order to help you be the author of your own valued directions, and to begin to pursue your valued aims, I have included the following worksheet. Allow yourself the time to complete the worksheet in a place that feels safe to you and where you will be free from interruptions. And then schedule another time a day or so later to look at your worksheet and reflect upon your answers.

Becoming the Author of My Valued Aims and Directions

This worksheet is intended to give you some space to write down some observations about what valued patterns of behaviour you would like to pursue in your life. Please take a few moments to complete each section, and reflect upon what aims you might pursue in your life that would be meaningful, rewarding and involve a sense of vitality and purpose for you.

1. Career

How important is this area of my life to me? (0-10): _____

What would my intention be in this area?

_____

_____

_____

_____

What obstacles might I face in realizing this intention?

_____

_____

_____

_____

How might I overcome these obstacles?

_____
_____
_____
_____

2. Family

How important is this area of my life to me? (0-10): _____

What would my intention be in this area?

_____
_____
_____
_____

What obstacles might I face in realizing this intention?

_____
_____
_____
_____

How might I overcome these obstacles?

_____
_____
_____
_____

3. Intimate Relationships

How important is this area of my life to me (0-10): _____

What would my intention be in this area?

_____
_____
_____
_____

What obstacles might I face in realizing this intention?

_____

_____

_____

_____

How might I overcome these obstacles?

_____

_____

_____

_____

4. Social Life

How important is this area of my life to me? (0-10): _____

What would my intention be in this area?

_____

_____

_____

_____

What obstacles might I face in realizing this intention?

_____

_____

_____

_____

How might I overcome these obstacles?

_____

_____

_____

_____

5. Education

How important is this area of my life to me? (0-10): _____

What would my intention be in this area?

_____

_____

_____

_____

What obstacles might I face in realizing this intention?

_____

_____

_____

_____

How might I overcome these obstacles?

_____

_____

_____

_____

6. Physical Well-Being

How important is this area of my life to me? (0-10): _____

What would my intention be in this area?

_____

_____

_____

_____

What obstacles might I face in realizing this intention?

_____

_____

_____

_____

How might I overcome these obstacles?

_____

_____

_____

_____

7. Spirituality

How important is this area of my life to me? (0-10): _____

What would my intention be in this area?

_____

_____

_____

_____

What obstacles might I face in realizing this intention?

_____

_____

_____

_____

How might I overcome these obstacles?

_____

_____

_____

_____

8. Community Involvement

How important is this area of my life to me? (0-10): _____

What would my intention be in this area?

_____

_____

_____

_____

What obstacles might I face in realizing this intention?

_____

_____

_____

_____

How might I overcome these obstacles?

_____

_____

_____

_____

9. Hobbies and Recreation

How important is this area of my life to me? (0–10): _____

What would my intention be in this area?

_____

_____

_____

_____

What obstacles might I face in realizing this intention?

_____

_____

_____

_____

How might I overcome these obstacles?

_____

_____

_____

_____

Reflecting upon Your Valued Aims and Planning for Compassionate Behaviour

After you have completed the worksheet and can take some time to reflect upon what you have learned, remember that a short exercise in a book like this isn't necessarily going to become the blueprint for a whole new life; however, it can be one step towards your gradual process of developing compassionate behaviour and mindfulness. When your behaviour becomes consistent with what you value, you are closer to living a life of compassion and on the way to being better able to face and overcome your fear and anxiety in the service of a life well lived. This might mean making some difficult decisions. For example, if you value physical well-being you may need to refrain from eating unhealthy foods that might taste good in the short term but which could pose a health risk to you. You might desire an extra glass of wine or two, but you might begin to forgo that kind of indulgence so that you may live a healthier and more productive life. Each of us is different, with a unique set of values, physical and emotional strengths and learning histories; however, we all have the capacity to cultivate our compassionate and mindful emotion-regulation system and to develop our compassionate selves through the many skills and attributes of our compassionate minds. An important part of that process is to face our fears in order to move towards what matters most to us.

Developing the Motivation to Face Your Fears

In this next section we'll look at the outline of a systematic plan for gradually facing your anxiety and for gradually exposing you to the experiences you would much rather avoid. In order to prepare for this, it is useful to enhance your compassionate motivation.

There are many reasons why we may experience problems with anxiety in our lives. Sometimes, our experience of anxiety seems clearly related to an ongoing psychological problem or 'anxiety disorder' and may include such compulsions as repeatedly checking the oven to see whether the gas has been switched off. At other times, stressful events in our lives such as unemployment, the breakup of a relationship or some other loss may increase our experience of anxiety. From the perspective of the compassionate mind, it is important to remember that the anxiety you experience is *not your fault*, that you didn't choose to have such an active threat-detection system, or the many reasons and causes for your struggle with anxiety. As much as you can, aim to have compassion for yourself, and acceptance of your anxiety, knowing that your suffering is a fundamental part of being human. Recognizing that this is a part of your essential humanity, and having sensitivity to that may help increase your motivation to face your fears, and move towards the life that you wish to live.

Do you have a paper and pen handy? If not, take a moment to find them, or your notebook that you've been keeping by your side. When you are ready, and have some uninterrupted time in your safe place, let's take a moment to recognize and reflect upon how much in life you may have given up because of anxiety. Jot down your answers to the following few questions:

- How much has your struggle with anxiety cost you in terms of your personal relationships? Have you avoided relationships, or have they become strained due to the limits your anxiety has placed upon you?

- Have you avoided things because of your anxiety and as a result missed out on financial, career or social opportunities? Have you made decisions that have had a negative impact on your work life or your financial life that have been based in anxiety?

- Has your struggle with anxiety limited the amount of freedom you have to pursue the things that you enjoy? Have you given up recreational activities, travel or hobbies due to avoidance behaviours?

- How much time and energy has been absorbed by negative emotions involved with your struggle with anxiety?

- What other things have you given up due to anxiety? What has anxiety cost you overall in your life?

As you answered these questions it is likely that you began to understand the impact that your anxiety has had on your life. The good news is that you are now taking steps to overcome this anxiety, and to take your life back. As we move towards the gradual exposure exercise it is important to remember your aim to reclaim your life and to free yourself to experience life with kindness, courage and authority. In engaging in exposure, you are going to be willingly experiencing some anxiety and distress in the short term so that you might better overcome anxiety in the long term.

Engaging in compassionate gradual exposure asks us to accept the fact that we may feel more anxiety before we feel less. By now we know that anxiety can arrive suddenly, and move through us to activate our physical sensations, emotions and thoughts. We also know that anxiety isn't easily controlled or suppressed and that the key is to meet it with compassionate courage and to be able to tolerate our distress. In CFT we often use the motto 'challenging but not overwhelming' to describe this gradual way of approaching anxiety.

With this in mind, let's use the chart set out below to record and examine the costs and benefits of engaging in compassionate gradual exposure. Let's imagine for a moment that I had a great fear of public speaking but a willingness to speak in public would be beneficial to my work as a psychologist, not only because of the need to lecture at university but also to give workshops and discuss research with groups of colleagues. So, if I had a phobia of public speaking it would probably be a good idea for me to aim to overcome it.

If I were to look at the costs and benefits of engaging in gradual exposure to this fear, I would probably list a number of costs. Firstly, engaging in the exposure would cause me to feel anxious, both at the time of exposure and in anticipation of it. If I were engaging in this with the help of a therapist I may also have to consider the cost of the therapy sessions and the cost in terms of time and effort. On the other hand, if I were to think about the benefits of engaging in gradual exposure, I would realize that if I overcame my anxiety and fears I would no longer be inclined to avoid situations where I would be required to speak in public. Additionally, this exposure might help me reduce my anxiety in a wide range of other situations over the course of my career and possibly make new opportunities available to me such as speaking at conferences and learning more from my colleagues, who I would be able to speak with more freely. So, even though there might have been some well-defined costs I can see how the benefits of engaging in this method of treatment would clearly outweigh them and that the act of engagement would be an exercise in compassion and courage.

In the table below, list the specific costs and benefits that you might face:

Costs of Facing My Fears	Benefits of Facing My Fears

What have you discovered after reviewing and listing the costs and benefits of gradual exposure? Have you created a clear vision in your mind of how your life would be improved by coping with your anxiety? You might want to review the list you made during chapter . . . to describe the ways that your life would be improved by your ability to cope with anxiety in a more mindful and compassionate way.

Exposure on a Gradual, Compassionate Path

The next steps show us how a compassionate gradual and systematic progress through a hierarchy of challenging experiences can help us overcome anxiety.

Take these exercises only as far as feels right to you and explore the possibility of working with a cognitive-behavioural therapist or support group for anxiety as you work through them if necessary. As we begin, let's clarify what we mean when we use the term exposure, which is a method of therapy that has been used for decades to help people overcome their fears by guiding them to remain in the presence of situations that cause them to experience elevated levels of anxiety. When we willingly remain close to what causes us fear, gradually fear can lose its power over our behaviour. How does this work?

Well, from a certain point of view, exposure works through a process known as 'habituation'. For a very long time, behaviour therapists assumed that when we remained in the presence of anxiety-provoking things for long enough, gradually our capacity to remain frightened in a given situation becomes exhausted. What tends to happen with people with anxiety is that rather than staying with the situation until the anxiety begins to subside and go away, they leave the situation while their anxiety is still building or intense. Or, they might think that because the thought of such a situation will make them anxious, they avoid it. But, as you and I have learned, this *can actually make things worse*. The reason is that when people briefly encounter an anxiety-provoking situation and then run away from it they only ever experience the intense, initial height of anxiety and never the experience of relief when it has subsided. This means that it is important to experience through compassionate mindfulness that anxiety doesn't exist as a permanent, endless state of affairs.

It may help to measure your own anxiety by grading it on a scale of 0–10, where 0 represents no anxiety at all and 10 the highest anxiety you could feel. This mindful process is sometimes referred to as a rating of 'Subjective Units of Distress' or SUD. Therapists often introduce anxiety-provoking images into their sessions as part of the process of gradually engaging in exposure, for example pictures of dogs if you have a fear of them. The therapist would then ask you what your SUD rating would be as you looked at a picture, which you would continue to do until your anxiety peaked (at whatever level, be it 4 or 5 or 6, et cetera) and until your feelings of anxiety then reduced by half. The therapist and you would decide how to gradually introduce more and more anxiety-provoking things into the situation week by week. For example, after looking at the picture of the dog you might watch a video of dog, then visit a pet store to see a dog in a cage. Gradually your exposure might involve approaching a dog, petting a puppy, or even playing with a fully grown Doberman. Your progress would depend on how much your anxiety decreased according to your SUD.

You may recall our discussion of desensitization, whereby we use our imagination to engage in and gradually decrease our experience of fear, panic and anxiety. This is similar to 'habituation'; however, something else is going on beyond the exhaustion of our ability to feel anxious. For one thing, we learn to be less frightened of being frightened; less anxious of being anxious. We begin to see that there are always going to be things that will make us anxious, such as taking exams, or a serious operation (either for ourselves or for someone we care for) or the need to find a new job. If we are able to tolerate our anxiety-related distress and accept that anxiety is a part of life then we also will be able to work with it and around it – in short, we will be better able to function in our lives.

In addition, it seems that when we remain in the presence of an anxiety-provoking situation long enough we have an opportunity to learn a range of new behaviours in response to that situation instead of just the 'fight, flight or freeze' mode of operating. Our practice of mindful and compassionate attention helps us to do this by giving us courage to face our fears. Remember, we learn to swim by being in the water, not just by reading the manual on how to do the backstroke.

The programme I've outlined below is based on years of research and development in CBT and CFT and can help you begin to work with exposure on your own – again, not just by reading through the steps but also by putting them in to practice. Additionally, I would highly recommend that you seek out a qualified CFT or CBT therapist to help you along the way.

Step One: What Triggers Your Fear?

When we engage in gradual exposure, the experience will depend on the focus of our fear (e.g., fear of flying, fear of dogs, fear of being in enclosed spaces) and the form of our avoidance behaviour (e.g., our fight, flight or freeze response).

To begin, it is important to identify and note down what your fears are, and what situations trigger elevated levels of anxiety for you; as you begin to think about your fears, please include the range of different situations and experiences in the outside world, and in your mind, that may trigger your threat-detection system.

To prepare, find a time when you can sit in your safe place without interruption for a while. When you are there, move into a grounded and stable seated posture as you do when you are practising mindfulness and compassionate imagery exercises. Start by taking a few soothing-rhythm breaths, emphasizing the exhale and then slowing the breathing down. Remind yourself that experiencing anxiety is a natural part of life, that it can be challenging and that your fears and worries are not your fault. Recognize that as you begin to list these fears in preparation for gradual exposure, you are engaging in a courageous and compassionate behaviour, and moving towards taking care of yourself as best as you can. These steps are meant to be 'challenging but not overwhelming'.

When you are ready, we will begin to use the form below to list the things that provoke your anxiety and fear. We will make two lists: the first will be of events 'outside' yourself – the situations, events, people and things that provoke problematic levels of anxiety for you. Feel free to list whatever comes to mind in this area and in whatever order. Let's look at an example of some of the situations that Jennifer, the client I introduced earlier, would have written down in such a list. Jennifer experienced panic attacks, some social anxiety, and had some persistent worries about approval and work performance. When her therapy with me began, panic attacks were on the top of her list, and her list of feared situations read something like this:

- riding on the subway

- speaking in front of class

- driving over the George Washington Bridge

- being in closed spaces

- meeting new people

- being in a crowded room

When you complete this step you might notice that just thinking about some of these things and writing them down can be a little anxiety provoking, can't it? This is completely natural, and is another example of how your 'always on, better-safe-than-sorry' threat-detection system is ready to fire up at a moment's notice in order to keep you safe. Take a moment though to realize that this is completely natural, and bring yourself back into the present, connecting with the rhythm of your breathing and holding yourself in kindness.

Your list might be very different because it will be unique to you. Here is the form you may use to create your first list of events 'outside' yourself that trigger your anxiety:

My Anxiety–Provoking and Feared Situations and Circumstances

The next list will involve those 'inside' events – the mental events, thoughts, images and physical sensations that provoke anxiety and represents those things 'inside' your mind that lead you into states of fear and worry. Many of these may seem to pop into your head all on their own or make you feel physically anxious without any prior warning, which in itself can provoke a great deal of anxiety. Just as we did with the list of 'outside' events, let's take a look at a few of the thoughts, emotions and images that Jennifer listed as she began her programme of gradual exposure:

- 'I am going to freak out'

- 'I can't handle it in here'

- 'I think I'm going to have a heart attack'

- 'I'm going to faint'

- 'I can't escape!'

- 'I'm going to freeze up in front of the class'

- picturing myself passed out on the floor of the train

- imagining myself being fired for not being able to speak in front of the class

- feeling nauseous

- feeling dizzy

- feeling 'closed in'

We can see a range of different anxiety-provoking thoughts that made their way on to Jennifer's list as well as the physical sensations that are related to panic attacks, and images that Jennifer identified as her 'inside' experiences that triggered her fear and anxiety. Now it's your turn again to use the form below to record your anxiety-provoking thoughts, sensations and inner experiences:

My Anxiety-Provoking Thoughts and Feared Inner Experiences

Many people describe how writing down their thoughts helps give them distance and perspective on their anxiety-provoking thoughts and inner dialogue. You might recall from the section on compassionate thinking that distancing and observing our anxiety-provoking and distressing mental events is an important step in developing a new and self-compassionate response system. This exercise is aimed at giving you similar distance so that you can observe your mental events with more flexibility, mindfulness and compassionate awareness and, in turn, help you move forward to develop a way to cope with your anxious suffering.

Step Two: What are Your Safety and Avoidance Behaviours?

As we have seen in our discussion of the nature of anxiety, we have evolved to respond to perceived threats with both an experience of anxiety and with avoidance behaviour. Understandably, avoiding real dangers in the outside world can be a life-saving strategy; however, it seems that problems arise when safety behaviours and avoidance strategies are used in response to our internal experiences of anxiety. Safety behaviours sometimes have unintended consequences, which may include a rise in anxiety-related behaviour in the long run, and missing out on valuable experiences in the present moment of our day-to-day lives. A safety strategy is something that is activated by our better-safe-than-sorry emotion-regulation system and it helps us only in the short term; so, how do we devise a strategy that can help us in the long term?

There is a substantial and compelling base of research that shows how efforts at suppressing distressing thoughts and avoiding emotional experiences can actually lead to an increase in the very thoughts and feelings were attempting to suppress.[5] I have seen this for myself when I've worked with clients who have struggled with their anxiety, and by my own experience of anxiety. The old adage that 'what we resist persists' really does seem to hold true. However, we can develop our compassionate minds to help us overcome our tendency towards unhealthy avoidance and give us courage to face what we fear. Think about it this way: a six-year-old child becomes anxious at the prospect of going to a friend's birthday party. There will be many people there from school but also many other children he won't know. His mother doesn't like to see him anxious and so tells him, 'Don't worry, you don't have to go. You can stay home with me.' She believes she's done the right thing to alleviate his distress; unfortunately, what the child learns is that anxiety is too much to face and can be avoided, and that this avoidance has its own reward – staying at home. The gap then widens between his ability to socialize and the other children, some of whom have been told they are going to the party regardless of their anxiety but that they 'will be OK once they get there. Think of all the cake and the goody bags! And anyway, I'll collect you in only a couple of hours – that's not too long, is it?' their mothers might say to encourage them. When they go, and face the possibility of anxiety, or the initial feelings of anxiety, they are learning to deal with their anxiety, and experience its subsidence as they begin to relax and make friends. Our shy child, on the other hand, feels reassured by being allowed to stay at home but he is not developing any of the skills needed to get on in the world and cope with his anxiety and develop his confidence. What do you think happens three weeks later when there's another party? Avoidance is not the same as compassion – the shy child's mother wants to be kind but she is operating in 'better-safe-than-sorry' mode; the compassionate mother knows the importance of not doing that, the importance of understanding and validating her child's feelings but also of finding a way to encourage her child.

The CFT approach helps us to encourage our own selves with reasoning, kindness, validation of our feelings and with compassion. When we practise imagining the compassionate self, for example, we give the compassionate self a sense of authority, wisdom and confidence, and it is these qualities that we aim to get in touch with so that we can experience the situations that are difficult for us.

As we begin to understand how we engage in safety behaviours and the many other forms of avoidance as we prepare for gradual exposure let's take a look again at Jennifer, whose avoidance and safety behaviours intensified her distress.

After having a panic attack on the subway, Jennifer became increasingly convinced that riding certain crowded trains would lead to intolerable levels of anxiety and panic. In response to her fear, she developed a range of safety behaviours she thought would help her avoid an emotional experience that she deemed impossible to bear: she kept one dose of anxiety medication in her purse 'in case she needed it' but would never take it; she always carried a full bottle of water on her commute to work 'in case she began to feel nauseous'; she took particular books with her on the train so that she could read familiar passages over and over again in order to distract herself; when she could, she would enlist a 'safety person' to ride the train with her; sometimes she took routes that were out of her way just so that she could travel on less crowded trains; additionally, she spent a great deal of money on taxis, or walked long distances to stay away from the possibility of having an anxiety attack on the subway.

When she did experience elevated high levels of anxiety or physical sensations that she associated with anxiety and panic, she would attempt to suppress these experiences, and chide herself for feeling as she did. This resulted in a cycle of intensifying anxiety.

As she and I began working on her compassionate gradual exposure, Jennifer took an inventory of her safety and avoidance behaviours and considered their unintended consequences. After a little while, it became clear that her attempts to ensure control and safety only reinforced her belief that she was in danger and strengthened her cycle of fear and panic. She also realized how much time and effort she was spending to carry out these behaviours – time and effort that could have been devoted to the pursuit of her valued aims and directions.

Just like Jennifer, we all have certain safety behaviours and patterns of avoidance that, despite their intention of 'safety', might not be helping us. With this in mind, let's use the form below to inventory your own safety behaviours and forms of avoidance.

In order to get a sense of what how this inventory is used, I've included an example of a completed form, listing safety behaviours and avoidance:

My Safety Behaviours and Forms of Avoidance
Taking taxis rather than riding on the subway
Carrying a bottle of water
Avoiding eye contact when speaking at work
Staying away from crowds
Avoiding bridges
Not attending parties and conferences
Having a 'safety person' with me whenever I travel or might become anxious

My Safety Behaviours and Forms of Avoidance

Step Three: Creating Your Fear Hierarchy

A fear hierarchy ranks your feared situations and events in order of how distressing they seem to you. Gradual exposure engagement often uses these hierarchies as tools that we can use to allow us to gradually increase our ability to remain in the presence of difficult experiences. Earlier, we made lists of events in the outside world and of our inner experience and situations that we might typically avoid. On the basis of these lists, and anything else that comes to mind, you will soon create a fear hierarchy of your own that you can use to engage in your own exposure exercises.

In the form below, list a range of situations and experiences that are connected to your fears and anxiety. Start off with the *least* anxiety-provoking circumstance and work your way up to those things that you find *most* anxiety provoking. As with the other written exercises, make sure you find a time to do this when you can be in your safe place and without interruption.

An example for your list might include something like: 'looking at a picture of an airplane' as your least anxiety-provoking circumstance if you have a fear of flying. This might seem rather mild but remember that even imaginary or pictorial representations of the things that provoke our anxiety can be effective in gradual exposure.

Some of the exposure exercises involve actual exposure to real-life situations; for example, eventually and when you are ready, real-life exposure might include actually being on a plane if you have a fear of flying. It won't necessarily mean taking off and flying – that might happen at a later stage, when you are ready – but it may mean stepping on to the plane, or on to the runway, et cetera, as gradually as is necessary. As you complete the fear hierarchy below, feel free to include the range of situations and experiences that provoke anxiety for you, whether or not it seems likely that you would engage in real-life exposure to them.

Included in the form is column for you to record your SUD ratings so that you can see how anxiety-provoking certain situations may be for you during your exposure exercises. In your fear hierarchy, I would like you to estimate the SUD that you imagine you would experience during exposure to each of these situations. This will help you to place the hierarchy in order, and plan your compassionate gradual exposure. In addition to this numerical assessment, feel free to jot down any other observations about how you imagine exposure to this anxiety-provoking situation might affect you.

Just like the form for safety behaviours and avoidance, below you will find an example of a completed hierarchy, and then a blank form for you to complete yourself.

My Fear Hierarchy			
Rank	Feared Situation or Experience	SUD 0–10	Observations
1	Being stuck in a subway car	10	'Don't think I could face it!'
2	Freezing during a presentation	8	
3	Being humiliated at an office party, saying something stupid	8	'Really afraid of the embarrassment'
4	Getting stuck on a bridge in a car	7	
5	Feeling crushed in a crowd	6	
6	Going on a first date	6	
7	Meeting people on a job interview	6	
8	Having a panic attack at work	5	'I would just feel out of control'

My Fear Hierarchy			
Rank	Feared Situation or Experience	SUD 0–10	Observations

Step Four: Prepare to Face Your Feared Situations

The CFT techniques and concepts we have explored will help you prepare for compassionate gradual exposure. It is important to remember that during these process we must remain in the presence of anxiety-provoking circumstances *without blocking or suppressing our anxiety*; however, it is also important to remember that when we practise *compassionate* gradual exposure we can call upon our mindful, compassionate self to give us courage and to hold us in warmth as we face our difficulty. In this way, we are accessing our compassionate emotion-regulation system by being kind to ourselves, by being willing, accepting, non-judgemental and wise in the knowledge that we are moving towards the pursuit of our valued aims.

As we prepare to engage in compassionate gradual exposure we may bring to mind the image of our compassionate ideal, and connect with the fact that life is difficult and presents us with many challenges, such as anxiety, which is neither our fault nor our enemy.

Although exposure involves deliberate contact with anxiety, we can remind ourselves that over the course of our lives we have encountered anxiety hundreds or thousands of times, sometimes on a daily basis, and sometimes so often that it has begun to rule our lives. We may often have found ourselves engulfed by the activity of our threat-detection system as we acted on autopilot. Now we have begun to understand that we can bring compassion to this realization, and deliberately adopt a non-judgemental acceptance of our experience. In preparation for compassionate gradual exposure, it may be helpful to ask what your compassionate self would say about your engagement in gradual exposure. You may even wish to place your hand or hands over your heart, deliberately directing loving kindness towards yourself, and connecting with a heartfelt desire to alleviate your struggle with anxious suffering.

It may also be helpful for you to visualize what it would be like to have completed a course of compassionate gradual exposure. What kind of new possibilities would present themselves to you after you have learned to cope with and manage your anxiety? Would you feel a sense of accomplishment for calling on your compassionate self to help you have the courage to face your fears?

Begin to prepare with your soothing-rhythm breathing. Find safe place during a time when you won't be interrupted and where you can sit comfortably, with the soles of your feet on the ground and with your back supported and straight. Let your tongue rest in your jaw and take a few mindful breaths. With your next natural exhale, begin to follow the steps set out below:

- Create an image of yourself going through first steps of compassionate gradual exposure.

- Acknowledge that the first steps are likely to be anxiety provoking.

- Bring to mind your compassionate self and imagine that self helping you engage with the anxiety-provoking situation.

- Focus on the feelings that you may have as you compassionately and gradually engage with the situation.

- See yourself coping with the situation, tolerating the anxiety, making contact with your breathing and using your mindful and compassionate thinking. Focus on the compassionate, validating and understanding voice that is within you.

- Remind yourself that the anxiety isn't permanent and will ebb and flow away.

- Walk yourself through the steps you will be taking and see yourself coping with them.

- See yourself coming through the anxiety and smiling to yourself with the pleasure of achievement.

This is the ideal situation; however, this is a difficult process and sometimes things don't always go according to plan or to how we've imagined them. If things get a bit more tricky, you can:

- Remember that things don't always go smoothly and that you are doing the best you can. It's similar to learning a new sport: sometimes you can see yourself improving but other times you feel stuck – this is all perfectly normal.

- As much as you can, return to the perspective of your compassionate self and remind yourself you can have another go at this on another day.

- Make sure you haven't tried to engage with something in your hierarchy that is perhaps is a bit too much at this stage; alternatively, try to find a way to adapt your exposure to adjust to a possible glitch.

- Always remain self-compassionate when things get difficult and when you hear the voice of your inner critic acknowledge its presence but then focus on your breathing and let the criticism go as you refocus on the compassionate gradual exposure.

  (You may find it helpful to write these points on a card or in your notebook that you can refer to again when things get tricky.)

Step Five: Engaging in Compassionate Gradual Exposure

We've now reached the point where you can begin to engage in compassionate gradual exposure to your anxiety. There are several ways of practising but we're going to focus on two methods that are well suited to treating a wide range of anxiety-based problems. The first method is known as 'imaginary' or 'imaginal' exposure, which involves the process of imagining that we are in the situation that we would fear. For example, if I were afraid of heights, I might imagine myself standing at the top of the Empire State Building, leaning over the guard rail on the observation deck, and looking down at the tiny street below from a dizzying height. Although this isn't as anxiety provoking as 'the real thing', it still makes my body and mind respond as if it were happening in real life. In this way, imaginary exposure can be quite anxiety provoking; therefore, it is an effective method of introducing us to compassionate gradual exposure.

The second method we will be practising is known as 'real-life exposure', when we actually face and engage with the situations and circumstances we have listed in our fear hierarchy. We won't be putting ourselves in situations that could cause us harm but we will be willingly entering into situations that cause us anxiety. So, if my fear were of heights and I were engaging in real-life exposure, I would purchase a ticket to the top of the Empire State Building, hop in the lift and actually stand on that observation deck rather than just imagining that I am doing so. As you would expect, truly facing the things that frighten us in real-life exposure can be challenging but it can also be a highly effective way to liberate us from our fears.

As you move up the fear hierarchy you are likely to experience greater levels of anxiety but this is part of the process of overcoming anxiety through compassionate gradual exposure, and as you engage in the exercise it is important that you recognize and let go of any safety or avoidance behaviours. As we have seen, these behaviours typically only help us in the short term and prevent us in the long term from pursuing our valued aims and directions. Letting go of these behaviours to fully engage with the process of exposure is a mindful act of courage and self-compassion.

Imaginary Exposure

In order to begin practising imaginary exposure, you'll need to find a time and a place where you can sit quietly without interruption and with your eyes closed for about ten to fifteen minutes. Based on the situations listed in your fear hierarchy, you are going to imagine scenarios in which you encounter your fears. You should begin with the least anxiety-provoking situation and gradually work your way through the more anxiety-provoking scenarios. Begin with your soothing-rhythm breathing – the soles of your feet are grounded, your posture is straight, comfortable and supported and you have allowed the hint of a smile to form. Your eyes remain closed but you are alert. After a few moments, begin to imagine the scenario that corresponds to the first item on your hierarchy. As vividly as you can, stay with this imaginary situation as if it were actually happening in the present moment. You may begin to feel some anxiety but it is important to resist the temptation to engage in any safety or avoidance behaviours. Every two minutes or so rate your SUD on a scale of 0-10. This will help you notice your distress increasing or decreasing depending on where you are in the engagement. Continue to run through your list for ten to fifteen minutes, or until your SUD rating reaches a peak of 10, and then drops to about half of that. This drop in SUD represents the process of habituation, which will help you become familiar with the feeling of anxiety and then also with relief once your anxiety begins to subside. The more often you do this the less anxiety-provoking this situation will be in the long term.

You should aim to practise this exercise daily until you feel familiar with, or habituated to, the feeling of anxiety provoked by each situation on the hierarchy, and the corresponding feeling of relief as the anxiety dissipates. You will gradually increase your exposure to anxiety-provoking situations on the hierarchy. Stay with the exposure for each situation until you believe you have habituated to it, a sensation that may even be indicated by feelings of boredom associated with what you've imagined. That is perfectly OK! Isn't it preferable to feel boredom when you are engaging with something you had previously feared or felt anxious about? As you become less anxious your attention can turn itself to other things and by doing so give you the opportunity to respond in new ways to things you had previously felt anxious about. In each stage of this process you are learning that you can face your fear and that your threat-detection system can set off false alarms that you don't need to obey. You are learning that you can engage with your anxiety but that you are in fact *choosing* to willingly stay with the image that frightens you. Once you feel ready, you can then choose to move on to the next item in your hierarchy until you have completed the range of anxiety-provoking scenarios that you have imagined and included on your list.

As you practise compassionate gradual exposure, it is a good idea to contact your compassionate self after each session. Throughout, you should stay with your stable posture, a kind half smile, closed eyes, and soothing-rhythm breathing. Drop into the present moment with the next natural inhale and bring the image of your compassionate self to mind. For a few moments, recognize what your compassionate self would say about your engagement with compassionate gradual exposure. Give yourself credit and appreciation for having the courage to turn towards those things that cause you fear in order to live your life more fully and follow in the direction of your valued aims.

It is important to engage in compassionate gradual exposure voluntarily, and at a pace that feels right to you. The process should be 'challenging but not overwhelming', not so difficult that it makes you distraught, discouraged and ready to give up trying. Remember to be kind to yourself, even as you face your fears.

The chart below is set out so that you can record your progress with compassionate general exposure using the imaginary method and includes the space for you to note down any observations that you wish to remember along the way.

My Imaginary Exposure Record Date:		
Feared Image:		
Time (in 2-minute intervals for SUD ratings)	SUD (0–10)	Observations (optional)

Here is an example of a completed record:

My Imaginary Exposure Record Date: 13 August 2012		
Feared Image: Being stuck for hours in a subway carriage without air conditioning		
Time (in 2-minute intervals for SUD ratings)	SUD (0–10)	Observations (optional)
1:58	8	This seems like it could be bad
2:00	9	
2:03	10	Very anxious now
2:06	10	Why am I doing this?
2:08	8	
2:10	7	OK, this is easing up a bit
2:12	6	
2:15	5	Getting used to it

Real-Life Exposure

After some time spent practising you may find that imaginary exposure has helped you begin to reduce the level of anxiety you experience when you think about the situations and events in your fear hierarchy. This is good news, represents progress. From here you may begin to engage in real-life exposure, the second method of compassionate gradual exposure. This follows a similar format to the imaginary method but this time you will be facing anxiety-provoking situations in the real world rather than in your imagination. It is important to recognize that you are not being asked to face situations that put you at risk of physical harm. The aim here is to bring ourselves into contact with situations that trigger intense levels of anxiety and fear, not to face dangerous situations.

Your compassionate gradual exposure will depend upon the type of anxiety you suffer from; for example, if you suffer from claustrophobic-related anxiety you may be begin to engage in exposure to an enclosed space such as phone booth. If you have a fear of having panic attacks in a crowded space then you may engage in compassionate gradual exposure to the hierarchy of fears on your list such as going to a sold-out sporting event or a popular museum exhibit.

Just as we did with imaginary exposure, while you are undergoing the exercise it may help you to record your SUD ratings every two minutes. Stay with the exposure until your SUD ratings peak and then drop by half. Again, it is important to take things gradually, and to be sensitive to your own limits. I like to tell my clients that they can work on the edge of their comfort zone, gradually stretching their capacity to tolerate distress and anxiety step by step. This can be a bit trickier with real-life exposure than it is with imaginary exposure, since real-life situations don't always correspond to brief or limited periods of time. For example, if I'm afraid of flying and am engaging in real-life exposure to a short flight, the most anxiety-provoking situation on my fear hierarchy list, I obviously won't be able to do that for ten or fifteen minutes as I had done with my imaginary method. So, we need to be sensitive to this, creative in our approach to practising real-life exposure, and willing and prepared to face life on its own terms. Working with our compassionate mind, and accessing our compassionate self can be very helpful in these situations, when they can give us the courage to face our anxiety and follow our valued aims and directions.

Additionally, many of my CFT clients have found it useful to create a series of 'coping statements', based upon compassionate thinking, in advance of entering into anxiety-provoking situations such as real-life exposure. These statements have traditionally been written on postcards of my clients' choosing, which we have called 'coping cards'. Recently, an increasing number of my clients have preferred to record these notes in an app on their mobile phones. In order to come up with some of these statements you might ask yourself what you would like to hear from a loving, strong and supportive friend who was walking alongside you as you engaged in your compassionate gradual exposure. What words of encouragement, support and authoritative helpfulness would help you to feel safe, resilient and ready to move forward in the face of fear, difficult emotions and anxiety? Below are a few examples of compassionate coping statements that may be helpful. Feel free to use these yourself but try also to come up with your own statements that are uniquely suitable to you:

- Anxiety is a natural part of life, and it makes sense that I would feel this way.

- I know these anxious feelings are unpleasant but I also know that am not in any danger. I can tell that these uncomfortable emotions and sensations are anxiety because they've been triggered by these predictable circumstances that I've begun to engage in.

- If this were a problem more serious than anxiety then it wouldn't come and go as it does.

I'd like you to think about these statements by closing your eyes for a moment, slowly breathing in and out. Bring to mind the sense of being a compassionate person and the image of your compassionate self, complete with a sense of wisdom and a genuine wish to be helpful, caring and warm. Now, open your eyes and read those statements again, but this time focus on their kindness and understanding. Don't worry if you believe them or not, or whether they are accurate or not, just focus on your emotions as you speak the words out loud.

Did you notice any difference? Here are some further coping statements to help you work from a compassionate, feeling perspective:

- Experiencing anxiety is *not my fault*; it's just a part of being human.

- Feelings are not facts.

- Emotions and responses like anxiety are not permanent; they will pass.

- This feeling will rise and fall and I can ride it like a wave until it dissipates.

- By facing this fear I'm opening myself up to living more fully and in the direction of my valued aims.

So, by willingly engaging in compassionate gradual exposure to real-life situations that make you anxious, and by responding to your anxiety with compassion, courage and wisdom, you are taking strong steps in compassionate behaviour that can lead you from a life dominated by anxiety to a life that is directed towards valued aims. The form will help you to keep track of your progress on the next page.

Taking Compassionate Exposure Further and Facing Fear in Everyday Life

The plan for gradual exposure that we have worked through is a structured way to face anxiety and overcome the hold anxiety has on your behaviour and your life; however, our ultimate aim is that the lessons

My Real–Life Exposure Record Date:		
Feared Image:		
Time (in 2-minute intervals for SUD ratings)	SUD (0–10)	Observations (optional)

of compassionate gradual exposure can be used in your everyday behaviour. A good way to practise this is by performing a 'behavioural experiment'. To do this, notice the anxiety-provoking situations you might have to engage with; then, when you do engage, you observe your anxiety response and carry on to complete your engagement with the situation.

Let's look at some examples of behavioural experiments in action. If I were a chronic worrier and heading out to the south of Spain for a holiday, my mind might generate a host of anxious predictions. I might pester myself with 'what ifs' such as, 'What if I get stuck in traffic and miss my flight?' or 'What if I get food poisoning?'; however, if I engaged in behavioural experiments I would notice my anxious prediction that I could get stuck in traffic, pause to validate and understand that prediction and then use compassionate attention to refocus my thoughts on the happy times I shall have on the holiday I have planned. After arriving at the airport, I might look back upon my worrisome predictions, and see how accurate they may have been, given that I left the house late and there was an accident en route. I might also notice that I was able to cope with the possibility of the delay by realizing that I hadn't left the house that late, that the accident was out of my control (and hope that no one was badly injured) and that my anxiety was not my fault. Regardless, so much of our suffering due to anxiety is due to worrisome predictions about things that never come to pass. As Mark Twain said, 'I am an old man and have known a great many troubles, but most of them never happened.' Often, when things do go wrong, we have far greater coping resources than our anxious minds allow us to believe we do, given that they are narrowly focused on the worry instead of the bigger picture. By cultivating our compassionate mind, we can engage in these behavioural experiments as often as seems workable while bringing mindful, compassionate behaviour, wisdom and courage into our everyday lives.

10 Moving Forward with Compassion and 'Beginning Again, Constantly'

> Having compassion starts and ends with having compassion for all those unwanted parts of ourselves, all those imperfections that we don't even want to look at. Compassion isn't some kind of self-improvement project or ideal that we're trying to live up to.
>
> Pema Chödrön, *When Things Fall Apart*

My own study and practice of psychology, compassionate mind training and mindfulness has been a deeply personal journey, as well as a professional mission.

We all share a common fate in our shared suffering, and my own unfolding history of loss, fear and trauma has taught me a great deal about what it means to approach my experience of anxiety with as much self-kindness, willingness and courage as I can, moment by moment. This isn't a process that reaches a point of completion. Every day there are new challenges, new worries and new encounters with emotional pain and doubt. Each moment presents an opportunity to return to a compassionate perspective, no matter how distressed we are. The English guitarist and expert on contemplative practice, Robert Fripp, has said, 'We begin again constantly.' I like this phrase – and remind myself of it when I practise the guitar and when I practise mindfulness and compassionate behaviour. It means that in this present moment, the only moment we will ever really experience, we can choose to make the decision to move forward in the direction of our valued aims – beginning now. This choice doesn't just pass us by to be lost for ever. It is a choice that is always available to us. We begin again and again, and our evolved capacity for compassion does not abandon us. It is available to us as we become available to it.

When I read new research and theories about meditation techniques or psychotherapy methods, I test them for myself as a matter of course. Ultimately, we all become our own therapists, our own scientists and our own guides, don't we? It would mean a great deal to me if you also did this for yourself when working with this book. Take *none* of what you have read on faith. Test each method. Explore and validate your own experience. We've looked at a number of ideas and techniques together, and this is the point of departure. Your completion of reading this book is a beginning, one that will see you engaging with these practices in ways that may help you overcome your struggle with anxiety, and move in valued directions.

As you do this, it is important to remember the often repeated idea that life is not about reaching a destination, but *is about the journey*. Your personal path, a life of mindful compassion, *is* your goal, and gently, consistently reminding yourself of this is a very good idea. Developing self-compassion isn't about perfecting yourself or finding a way to reach the top of the mountain; it is about accepting who you are, here and now, in this very moment.

I can clearly remember an evening I spent with warm and wise friends in Boston during the last few weeks of my internship year. I was filled with daydreams, plans and ambitions about where my life was headed, and how good things were going to be when I finally arrived at my destination. My attention and steady stream of chatter were all about how good it was going to be in the future, and how much happier I would be if I became someone new, someone more successful.

Meg, one of my friends who was there, took me by the hand for a moment, looked me in the eyes, and said, 'It's great to hear about all of your plans, Dennis, but I want you to remember that your life is happening right now. This *is* your life. It has already begun, and we are all here together and right now you are already good enough, just as you are, and we love you.' This kind of stopped me in my tracks. I felt very moved and filled with gratitude. I had been so fired up about the possibility for personal transformation and professional development that I couldn't really appreciate the joy and care that was present all around me that night. Of all of the different evenings I've spent with colleagues and buddies, this one often comes to mind. When I think of Meg's words, part of me feels nostalgic for that time in my life, but even that sort of misses the point. Meg was inviting me to show up to my life with compassionate acceptance, in contact with the present moment. Getting pulled into the future or lost in the past is very different to that idea. Right here and right now is where we live our lives. So, as you practise the development of your compassionate mind, my wish for you is that you can come into contact with the loving kindness, courage, warmth and wisdom that you already possess, and open yourself up to accepting yourself exactly as you are, in this very moment.

Throughout this book, we have learned that anxiety is a natural part of our human experience, that our 'always on, better-safe-than-sorry' threat-detection system has evolved as an essential part of our survival to help our species flourish. We understand that anxiety affects many aspects of us such as our thoughts, emotions and physical sensations. We have seen that when our threat-detection system is active and dominant, it uses our 'threatened mind' to influence our attention, thinking, motivations, emotions, imagination and our behaviour. We understand now that we have evolved to have a powerful capacity to feel fear and to protect ourselves by seeking safety, whether in the company of others or by fleeing a situation altogether. As important as this threat-detection system is, we know that the experience of intense and excessive anxiety can be distressful and can hold us back from fully experiencing our lives.

It is important for us to remember that our anxious suffering is not our fault. After all, each of us just finds ourselves here, emerging from the evolutionary flow of life on this planet. And, what we think and feel is related to our genetic history, and our learning history. We know that we didn't choose to have such tricky brains, but we also know that these allow us to use our learning histories, and the range of our personal circumstances, even traumatic events, to deal with, yet sometimes perpetuate our troubles with anxiety.

Thankfully, our rapid-response threat-detection system is not our only response system. Our tricky brains have evolved to let us reflect, develop long-term plans and observe our experiences from a flexible perspective, with wisdom and without judgement. Still more importantly, we have learned that experiencing compassion for ourselves and for others can be one of the most useful tools to help us overcoming our difficulties with anxiety and that kindness, warmth and a deep sensitivity to suffering in ourselves and others can begin to affect how we cope with our anxiety. CFT is based on the fact that the more we cultivate our capacity for compassion, the more we will activate our supportive and positive feelings involving the experience of safety, contentment and a secure base from where we can explore our world. As these feelings and alternate response systems are strengthened and activated more consistently, we can become more mindful, and more in touch with our compassionate selves.

Let's look now at a few ideas and simple steps that can help you continue the cultivation of your compassionate mind in order to overcome your struggle with anxiety. There are many ways that you can approach the material from this book, and the following steps suggest a path that may strengthen your practice, and provide you with some structure along the way.

Steps in Moving Forward (and Beginning Again, Constantly!)

1   Accept that anxious suffering is a part of the human condition

This is a point that we have looked at often, yet I feel that it remains important to outline the steps that you can take to bring compassion to your anxiety. 'The first noble truth of the Buddha is that when we feel suffering, it doesn't mean that something is wrong. What a relief. Finally somebody told the truth. Suffering is a part of life, and we don't have to feel it's happening because we personally made the wrong move.[1]

2   Gradually build your capacity for mindfulness

Mindfulness may not be an end in itself, but it can be an important part of our development of compassion, wisdom and courage. As we grow in our ability to remain in contact with the present moment, willingly and non-judgementally, we may loosen the grip that our anxious thoughts and feelings can have upon our minds and our behaviour. Thousands of years of Eastern meditative tradition as well as advanced Western scientific research have demonstrated how useful mindfulness can be as it helps us overcome our problems with anxiety. The mindfulness exercises in this book can serve as a structure for a daily practice. With consistent, engaged mindfulness practice our capacity to bring mindfulness to our everyday experience, moment by moment, can grow. You will develop an important new strength even if you begin by practising mindfulness for just a few minutes each day. In time, you may build a personal mindfulness practice that involves formal mindfulness training for twenty minutes each day or more. This can be a powerful ally for your work with anxiety, and the development of your compassionate mind. There are links to many resources for continuing your mindfulness practice, and several guided mindfulness meditations that are available for download at my website www.mindfulcompassion.com.

3   Use compassionate imagery

Your mind's ability to create an imaginary inner world, and to respond to this world with real emotions and behavioural changes, is a powerful tool for your compassionate mind training. Planning to spend some time each day practising compassionate imagery will help you access self-compassion when you need it. You can practise the longer, structured compassionate imagery exercises such as 'The Compassionate Self' exercise or 'The Compassionate Ideal' whenever you need to. When you sense feelings of anxiety building up, and may begin to feel overwhelmed, aim to contact the part of you that is supportive, helpful, encouraging and non-judgemental. This can help you experience anxiety from a secure base, without being engulfed in the anxiety, and feeling completely caught up in your fears.

4.   Return to compassionate thinking

When our anxious mind is activated, our attention can become narrower, our range of responses seem limited and our thinking threat-focused, worried and fearful; however, when we activate our compassionate mind we are providing ourselves with the opportunity to see things from a compassionate perspective and to realize how much of our lives we have given up to anxious thinking. When we do this, we can then choose to learn to use our compassionate reasoning to frame new responses that are more in tune with our capacity for warmth, wisdom and resiliency. The range of compassionate alternative responding techniques I have described are designed to help you practise this, and to help you take back control from worry, fear and panic. The compassionate-thought record and daily practice of compassionate thinking exercises can help us integrate compassionate responses into our everyday, automatic patterns of reacting to anxiety and a gradual, step-by-step engagement can help you build a bridge between a life dominated by anxiety, and a life where compassionate action becomes possible.

5.   Set your course, face your fears, and live a life of compassionate behaviour

We have evolved to seek safety and comfort through affiliation and to find a secure base from where we can explore the world. Affiliation helps us regulate our emotions and, as a result, to pursue our valued aims. Similarly, the development of mindful and compassionate attention, compassionate imagery and compassionate thinking provides a platform of compassionate wisdom that can allow you to build a life worth living. Anxiety can be distressful but it can also limit our prospects when we avoid certain situations that we fear, engage in hours of worry or compulsive behaviour and spend lost time engaging in safety behaviours. At times, it seems that anxiety and avoidance can become the organizing principles for how we approach our life. Compassionate behaviour involves taking action to identify the way we wish to change this so that we can cope with our anxiety, broaden our perspectives and prospects, clarify our valued aims and face our fears so that we may live more fulsomely. One of the most compassionate things we can do is to become sensitive to suffering and committed to taking action to alleviate that suffering in ourselves and others. Mindful, compassionate gradual exposure to our anxiety is a powerful example of a difficult but worthwhile exercise that can help liberate us from anxiety in the long term. Additionally, as your capacity for compassion grows, you may wish to expand your circle of compassionate behaviour by bringing your compassionate self into your life, for example as an active member of your community, as a family member, or as a partner in a personal or working relationship. As your heart opens in warmth and loving kindness to the common humanity of our anxious struggles, compassionate behaviour towards others, as well as yourself, is a powerful tool for living a bigger, more meaningful life.

'The Golden Rule': First, Inversion

As we reach the end of this book about compassion and anxiety, I'd like to acknowledge that there has been a bit of a paradox throughout these pages. We know that anxiety causes us to be fearful of what may happen to *us*, and involves a lot of inward-looking focus; however, compassion, when we read about it or talk about it, usually refers to a focus on others. Compassion is usually referred to in the context of how we are moved by the suffering of others, and how we act to help alleviate their suffering.

This is a powerful and important part of contacting our essential humanity, and will help us live mindfully and alleviate our own suffering.

In this book I've chosen to focus on how you might develop compassion for yourself and choose to direct your compassionate mind inward so that it can help you cope with your inward-focused anxiety. This choice partly reflects what I refer to as 'The Golden Rule: First, Inversion'. 'The Golden Rule', as it is popularly known, means that we should treat others as we would treat ourselves; however, this assumes that we treat ourselves well, and with kindness.[2] I'm afraid that we can't make this assumption. The epidemic levels of anxiety disorders, depression laced with worry and the general culture of fear and pressure for material success that surrounds us can drag us into a place of shame, self-criticism and neglect for our own well-being. Perhaps, as my colleague Chris Germer suggested, a new 'Golden Rule' should be called for, one that directs us to treat ourselves the way we would wish to be treated by others. I like to think of this as an inversion of the Golden Rule, which serves as a reminder of how we might begin again and again to hold ourselves in kindness and access our compassionate self.

This resonates with the aims of CFT, which helps us learn that compassion comes from within us but extends to others as we seek to address the suffering that we encounter in the wider world: 'The whole idea of compassion is based on a keen awareness of the interdependence of all these living beings, which are all part of one another, and all involved in one another.'[3]

I send my warmest wishes to you as you continue on your journey to cultivate your compassionate mind. Please feel free to contact me through my website.

Namaste.

DT

Notes

Preface

1 Dykas, M. J., & Cassidy, J., 'Attachment and the Processing of Social Information across the Life Span: Theory and Evidence', *Psychological Bulletin*, 137(1), (2011) 19–46.

   Gilbert, P., *The Compassionate Mind: A new Approach to Life's Challenges* (London: Constable Robinson, 2009).

2 Neff, K. D., Kirkpatrick, K., & Rude, S. S., 'Self-compassion and Its Link to Adaptive Psychological Functioning', *Journal of Research in Personality*, 41 (2007), 139–54.

3 Gilbert, P., & Procter, S., 'Compassionate Mind Training for People with High Shame and Self-Criticism: A Pilot Study of a Group-Therapy Approach', *Clinical Psychology and Psychotherapy*, 13, (2006) 353–79.

   Van Dam, N., Sheppard, S. C., Forsyth, J. C., & Earleywine, M., 'Self-Compassion Is A Better Predictor than Mindfulness of Symptom Severity and Quality of Life in Mixed Anxiety and Depression', *Journal of Anxiety Disorders*, 25, (2011), 123–30.

A Personal Story and Acknowledgements

1 Hayes, S. C., Stroshal, K. D., & Wilson, K. G., *Acceptance and Commitment Therapy: An Experiential Approach to Behavior Change* (New York: Guilford, 2009).

2 Linehan, M. M., *Cognitive Behavioral Treatment of Borderline Personality Disorder*. (New York: Guilford, 1993).

3 Leahy, R. L., Tirch D., & Napolitano, L., *Emotion-Regulation in Psychotherapy: A Practitioner's Guide* (New York: Guilford, 2011).

4 Gilbert, P., McEwan, K., Matos, M., & Rivis, A., 'Fears of Compassion: Development of Three Self-Report Measures', *Psychology and Psychotherapy*. (2011) [Epub ahead of print.]

5   Gilbert, P., *The Compassionate Mind: A New Approach to Life's Challenges* (London: Constable and Robinson, 2009).

Longe, O., Maratos, F. A., Gilbert, P., Evans, G., Volker, F., Rockliff, H., & Rippon, G., 'Having A Word with Yourself: Neural Correlates of Self-Criticism and Self-Reassurance', *Neuroimage*, 49 (2), (2010), 1849–56.

Chapter 1: The Emergence of Anxiety

1   Eysenck, M. W., Derakshan, N., Santos, R., & Calvo, M. G., 'Anxiety and Cognitive Performance: Attentional Control Theory', *Emotion, 7*, (2007), 336–53.

2   Hirschfeld, R. M. A., 'The Comorbidity of Major Depression and Anxiety Disorders: Recognition and Management in Primary Care', *Primary Care Companion: Journal of Clinical Psychiatry*, 3, (2001), 244–54.

3   Harter, M. C., Conway, K. P., & Merikangas, K. R., 'Association between Anxiety Disorders and Physical Illness', *European Archives of Psychiatry and Clinical Neuroscience*, 6, (2003), 313.

4   These statistics, and much more information about anxiety can be found at www.adaa.org/about-adaa/press-room/facts-statistics (ADAA, 2011).

5   Kessler, R. C. & Ustun, T. B., *The WHO World Mental Health Surveys* (Cambridge: Cambridge University Press, 2008).

6   Greenberg, P. E., Sisitsky, T., Kessler, R. C., et. al., 'The Economic Burden of Anxiety Disorders in the 1990s', *Journal of Clinical Psychiatry*, 60, (1999), 427–35.

Chapter 2: What is Anxiety and How Has it Evolved?

1   Hayes, S. C., Stroshal, K. D., & Wilson, K. G., *Acceptance and Commitment Therapy: An experiential Approach to Behavior Change* (New York: Guilford, 1999)

2   A point made by Professor A. T. Beck from the University of Pennsylvania, the founder of Cognitive Therapy.

3   Cook, M. & Mineka, S., 'Observational Conditioning of Fear to Fear-Relevant

Versus Fear-Irrelevant Stimuli in Rhesus Monkeys', *Journal of Abnormal Psychology*, 98 (1989), 448–59.

4 Ferster, C. B., 'A Functional Analysis of Depression', *American Psychologist*, 28 (1973), 857–70.

5 Hayes, S. C., Stroshal, K. D., & Wilson, K. G., *Acceptance and Commitment Therapy: An Experiential Approach to Behavior Change* (New York: Guilford, 2009).

Chapter 3: Anxiety, Compassion and Our Ongoing Interactions with the World

1 Gilbert, P., *The Compassionate Mind: A New Approach to Life's Challenges* (London: Constable and Robinson, 2009).

2 Goodall, J., *Through a Window: Thirty Years with the Chimpanzees of Gombe* (London: Penguin, 1990)

Chapter 4: Towards the Compassionate Mind: An Evolution in Our Understanding of Anxiety through Mindfulness, Acceptance and Compassion

1 Brownstein, M. J., 'A Brief History of Opiates, Opioid Peptides, and Opioid Receptors', *Proceedings of the National Academy of Science*, 90, (1993), 5391–3.

2 Possehl, G., *The Indus Civilization: A Contemporary Perspective* (Lanham, Maryland: AltaMira Press, 2003).

3 Deikman, A., *The observing self: Mysticism and Psychotherapy.* (Boston: Beacon Press, 1982).

4 Beck, A.T., *Cognitive Therapy and the Emotional Disorders* (New York: International Universities Press, 1976).

Ellis, A. & Dryden, W., *The Practice of Rational Emotive Behavior Therapy* (New York: Springer Publishing, 2007).

5 Kabat-Zinn, J., *Full Catastrophe Living* (New York: Delta Publishing, 1990).

6 Hayes, S. C., Stroshal, K. D., & Wilson, K. G., *Acceptance and Commitment Therapy: An Experiential Approach to Behavior Change* (New York: Guilford, 2009).

7 Hofmann, S. G., Sawyer, A. T., Witt, A. A., & Oh, D., 'The Effect of Mindfulness-Based Therapy on Anxiety and Depression: A Meta-Analytic Review', *The Journal of Consulting and Clinical Psychology*, 78, (2010). 169–83.

Baer, R. A., 'Mindfulness Training as a Clinical Intervention: A Conceptual and Empirical Review', *Clinical Psychological Science and Practice*, 10, (2003), 125–43.

8 Roemer, L. & Orsillo, S. M., 'An Open Trial of an Acceptance-Based Behavior Therapy for Generalized Anxiety Disorder', *Behavior Therapy*, 38, (2007), 78–82.

Roemer, L., Orsillo, S. M., & Salters-Pedneault, K., 'Efficacy of an Acceptance-Based Behavior Therapy for Generalized Anxiety Disorder: Evaluation in a Randomized Controlled Trial', *Journal of Consulting and Clinical Psychology*, 76, (2008), 1083–9.

9 H. H. Dalai Lama, *Transforming the Mind* (New York: Thorsons, 2000).

10 This quote is from an interview that can be found at: www.6seconds.org/modules.php?name=News&file=article&sid=260.

11 Mikulincer, M., & Shaver, P. R., *Attachment in Adulthood: Structure, Dynamics and Change* (New York: Guilford, 2007).

12 Gillath, O., Shaver, P. R., & Mikulincer, M., 'An Attachment-Theoretical Approach to Compassion and Altruism', in P. Gilbert (ed.), *Compassion: Conceptualisations, Research, and Use in Psychotherapy* (London: Brunner-Routledge, 2005).

13 Uvans-Moberg, K., 'Oxytocin May Mediate the Benefits of Positive Social Interaction and Emotions', *Psychoneuroendocrinology*, 23, (1998), 819–35.

Kosfeld, M., Heinrichs, M., Zak, P. J., Fischbacher, U., & Fehr, E., 'Oxytocin Increases Trust in Humans', *Nature*, 435, (2005), 673–6.

14 Lutz, A., Brefcyznski-Lewis, J., Johnstone, T., & Davidson, R. J., 'Regulation of the Neural Circuitry of Emotion by Compassion Meditation: Effects of Meditative Expertise', *Public Library of Science*, 3, (2008), 1–5.

15   LeDoux, J., *The Emotional Brain* (London: Weidenfeld & Nicolson, 1998).

16   Ibid.

17   Gilbert, P., *The Compassionate Mind: A New Approach to Life's Challenges* (London: Constable and Robinson, 2009).

   Gilbert, P., McEwan, K., Mitra, R., Franks, L., Richter, A., & Rockliff, H., 'Feeling Safe and Content: A Specific Affect Regulation System? Relationship to Depression, Anxiety, Stress and Self-criticism', *The Journal of Positive Psychology*, 3, (2008), 182–91.

18   Panskepp, J., *Affective Neuroscience* (New York: Oxford Press, 1998).

   Depue, R. A., & Morrone-Strupinsky, J.V., 'A Neurobehavioural Model of Affiliative Bonding', *Behavioral and Brain Sciences*, 28, (2005), 313–95.

19   Gilbert, P., *The Compassionate Mind: A New Approach to Life's Challenges* (London: Constable and Robinson, 2009).

20   Wang, S., 'A Conceptual Framework for Integrating Research Related to the Physiology of Compassion and the Wisdom of Buddhist Teachings' in P. Gilbert (ed.), *Compassion: Conceptualisations, Research and Use in Psychotherapy* (New York: Routledge, 2005).

21   Armstrong, K., *The Great Transformation: The World in the Time of Buddha, Socrates, Confucius and Jeremiah* (London: Atlantic Books, 2006).

22   Gilbert, P., *The Compassionate Mind: A New Approach to Life's Challenges* (London: Constable and Robinson, 2009).

23   Jung, C. G., 'The Archetypes and the Collective Unconscious', in *Collected Works of C. G. Jung*, Vol. 9, Part 1 (New Jersey: Princeton University Press, 1934).

24   Armstrong, K., *The Great Transformation: The World in the Time of Buddha, Socrates, Confucius and Jeremiah* (London: Atlantic Books, 2006).

25   Neff, K., *Self-Compassion: Stop Beating Yourself Up and Leave Insecurity Behind* (New York: Harper Collins, 2011).

   Neff, K. D., Kirkpatrick, K., & Rude, S. S., 'Self-Compassion and Its Link to Adaptive Psychological Functioning', *Journal of Research in Personality*, 41, (2007), 139–54.

26 Seigel, D. J., *The Mindful Brain* (New York: Norton, 2007).

27 Rahula, W., *What the Buddha Taught* (New York: Grove Press, 1959).

28 Lutz, A., Brefcyznski-Lewis, J., Johnstone, T., & Davidson, R. J., 'Regulation of the Neural Circuitry of Emotion by Compassion Meditation: Effects of Meditative Expertise', *Public Library of Science*, 3, (2008) 1–5.

29 Chödrön, P., *Start Where You Are: A Guide to Compassionate Living* (Boston: Shambhala, 2003).

Chapter 5: The First Turning of the Wheel of Compassion: Exploring the Attributes and Skills of the Compassionate Mind

1 Leahy, R. L., Tirch, D., Napolitano, L., *Emotion Regulation in Psychotherapy: A Practitioner's Guide* (New York: Guilford, 2011).

Tirch, D. D., & Leahy, R. L., 'Anxiety and Our Relationship to Emotional Experience: The Role of Emotional Schemas, Psychological Flexibility and Mindfulness'. Paper presented at the International Congress of Cognitive Psychotherapy, Istanbul (June, 2011).

Tirch, D. D., Leahy, R. L., & Silberstein, L. 'Relationships among Emotional Schemas, Psychological Flexibility, Dispositional Mindfulness, and Emotion Regulation'. Paper presented at the meeting of the Association for Behavioral and Cognitive Therapies, New York (November, 2009).

Chapter 6: Mindfulness as a Foundation for Compassionate Attention

1 Alan Watts is an extremely important and famous philosopher and writer on East/West philosophy, Zen and Vedanta from the UK in the late 1960s and early 1970s. He is a fantastic thinker and has recorded some wonderful lectures. I'd recommend checking him out.

Watts, A., *The Wisdom of Insecurity* (New York: Vintage: 1968).

2   Kabat-Zinn, J., *Full Catastrophe Living* (New York: Delta Publishing, 1990).

3   Kabat-Zinn, J., Foreword, in Didonna, F., (ed.), *Clinical Handbook of Mindfulness* (New York: Springer, 2009).

Siegel, R., Germer, C. K., & Olendzki, A., 'Mindfulness: What is it? Where did it come from?' in Didonna, F., (ed.), *Clinical Handbook of Mindfulness* (New York: Springer, 2009).

4   Wallace, B.A., 'A Mindful Balance', *Tricycle*, Spring 60–63 (2008), 109–11.

5   This excercise is adapted from, Gilbert, P., *The Compassionate Mind* (London: Constable & Robinson, 2009).

6   Davidson, R. J., Kabat-Zinn, J., Schumacher, J., Rosenkranz, M., Muller, D., et. al., 'Alterations in Brain and Immune Function Produced by Mindfulness Meditation', *Psychosomatic Medicine*, 65, (2003), 564–70.

Goldin, P. R., & Gross, J. J., 'Effects of Mindfulness-Based Stress Reduction (MBSR) on Emotion Regulation in Social Anxiety Disorder', *Emotion*, 10, (2010), 83–91.

7   This excercise has been adapted from multiple sources, including: Kabat-Zinn, J., *Wherever You Go, There You Are*: *Mindfulness Meditation in Everyday Life* (New York: Hyperion, 1994), and Leahy, R. L., Tirch, D., Napolitano, L., *Emotion Regulation in Psychotherapy: A Practitioner's Guide* (New York: Guilford, 2011).

8   This exercise was developed by two pioneers in the application of mindful compassion to psychotherapy, Dr Kristin Neff and Dr Christopher Germer, and appears in Dr Germer's book *The Mindful Path to Self-Compassion* (New York: Guilford Press, 2009).

9   Adapted from Leahy, Tirch and Napolitano, *Emotion Regulation in Psychotherapy: A Practitioner's -Guide* (New York: Guilford, 2011). This exercise is adapted from the MBCT protocol, cf., Segal, Z. V., Williams, J. M. G., & Teasdale, J. D., *Mindfulness-Based Cognitive Therapy for Depression: A New Approach to Preventing Relapse* (New York: Guilford, 2002).

10   Adapted from Leahy, Tirch and Napolitano, *Emotion Regulation in Psychotherapy: A Practitioner's Guide* (New York: Guilford, 2011).

11   Kamalashila, *Meditation: The Buddhist Way of Tranquillity and Insight* (Birmingham, England: Windhorst, 1992).

Chapter 7: Compassion-Focused Imagery

1 All of the compassionate imagery exercises have been adapted from CFT exercises found in Gilbert, P., *The Compassionate Mind* (London: Constable & Robinson, 2009), and other, unpublished CFT sources.

Chapter 8: Compassionate Thinking

1 Neff, K., *Self-Compassion: Stop Beating Yourself Up and Leave Insecurity Behind* (New York: Harper Collins, 2011).

2 Gilbert, P., *The Compassionate Mind: A New Approach to Life's Challenges* (London: Constable and Robinson, 2009).

3 Adapted from an exercise from Hayes, S. C., Stroshal, K. D., & Wilson, K. G., *Acceptance and Commitment Therapy: An Experiential Approach to Behavior Change* (New York: Guilford, 1999). Also found in variations in other sources throughout the ACBS community, cf. www.contextualpsychology.org.

Chapter 9: Compassionate Behaviour

1 Robb, H. From a personal communication by email (2010).

2 Dimidjian, S., Hollon, S. D., Dobson, K. S., Schmaling, K. B., Kohlenberg, R. J., Addis, M. E., Gallop, R., McGlinchey, J. B., Markley, D. K., Gollan, J. K., Atkins, D. C., Dunner, D. L., & Jacobson, N. S., 'Randomized Trial of Behavioral Activation, Cognitive Therapy, and Antidepressant Medication in the Acute Treatment of Adults with Major Depression', *Journal of Consulting and Clinical Psychology*, 74(4), (2006), 658–70.

3 Bennett-Levy, J., 'Mechanisms of Change in Cognitive Therapy: The Case of Automatic Thought Records and Behavioural Experiments', *Behavioural and Cognitive Psychotherapy*, 31, (2003), 261–77.

4 Hayes, S. C., Luoma, J., Bond, F., Masuda, A., & Lillis, J., 'Acceptance and Commitment Therapy: Model, Processes, and Outcomes', *Behaviour Research and Therapy*, 44(1), (2006), 1–25.

Hayes S. C., from a plenary talk at the 2008 conference of the Association for Behavioral and Cognitive Therapies, which can be viewed here: www.globalpres.com/mediasite/Viewer/?peid=017fe6ef4b1544279d8cf27adbe92a51.

5 Wenzlaff, R. M. & Wegner, D. M., 'Thought Suppression', *Annual Review of Psychology*, 51 (2000), 59–91.

Chapter 10: Moving Forward with Compassion and 'Beginning Again, Constantly'

1 Chödrön, P., *When Things Fall Apart* (Boston: Shambhala, 1997).

2 Germer, C., *The Mindful Path to Self-Compassion* (New York: Guilford Press, 2009).

3 Thomas Merton (1915–68) was a writer and a Trappist monk who encouraged interfaith understanding and was famous for gently integrating Buddhist and Christian philosophy in his work.

Further Resources

Books, Chapters and Articles

Barlow, D., *Anxiety and Its Disorders* (New York: Guilford, 2002).

Baer, R. A., 'Mindfulness Training as a Clinical Intervention: A Conceptual and Empirical Review', *Clinical Psychological Science and Practice*, 10, (2003) 125–43.

Brach, T., *Radical Acceptance: Embracing Your Life with the Heart of a Buddha* (New York: Bantam, 2004).

Cahn, B. R., & Polich, J., 'Meditation States and Traits: EEG, ERP, and Neuroimaging Studies', *Psychological Bulletin*, 132, (2006), 180–211.

Carter, C. S., 'Neuroendocrine Perspectives on Social Attachment and Love', *Psychoneuroendocrinology*, 23, (1998), 779–818.

Chödrön, P., *When Things Fall Apart: Heart Advice for Difficult Times* (Boston: Shambhala, 1997).

Chödrön, P., *Start Where You Are: How to Accept Yourself and Others* (London: Element/HarperCollins, 2005).

Cozolino, L., *The Neuroscience of Human Relationships: Attachment and the Developing Brain* (New York: Norton, 2007).

Craske, M. G., Kircanski, K., Zelikowsky, M., Mystkowski, J., Chowdhury, N. & Baker, A., 'Optimizing Inhibitory Learning During Exposure Therapy', *Behavior Research Therapy*, 46, (2008), 5–27.

Dalai Lama, *The Power of Compassion* (India: HarperCollins: 1995).

Dalai Lama, *An Open Heart: Practicing Compassion in Everyday Life* (New York: Little, Brown, 2001).

Dalai Lama & Cutler, H., *The Art of Happiness: A Handbook for Living* (New York: Riverhead Books, 1998).

Dalai Lama & Ekman, P., *Emotional Awareness: Overcoming the Obstacles to Psychological Balance and Compassion* (New York: Henry Holt & Co, 2008).

Davidson, R., & Harrington, A. *Visions of Compassion: Western Scientists and Tibetan Buddhists Examine Human Nature* (Oxford: Oxford University Press, 2002).

Depue, R. A., & Morrone-Strupinsky, J. V., 'A Neurobehavioural Model of Affiliative Bonding', *Behavioral and Brain Sciences*, 28, (2005), 313–95.

Farb, N. A. S., Segal, Z., Mayberg, V., Bean, H. J., McKeon, D., Fatima, Z., et al., 'Attending to the Present: Mindfulness Meditation Reveals Distinct Neural Modes of Self-Reference', *Social Cognitive Affective Neuroscience Advance Access*, 2, (2007), 1–10.

Germer, C. K., *The Mindful Path to Self-Compassion: Freeing Yourself from Destructive Thoughts and Emotions* (New York: The Guilford Press, 2009).

Gilbert, P., *The Compassionate Mind* (London: Constable and Robinson, 2009).

Gilbert, P., *Compassion Focused Therapy: Distinctive Features* (London: Routledge, 2010).

Gilbert, P., *Human Nature and Suffering* (London: Lawrence Erlbaum Associates, 1989).

Gilbert, P., McEwan, K., Mitra, R., Franks, L. Richter, A., & Rockliff, H., 'Feeling Safe and Content: A Specific Affect Regulation System? Relationship to Depression, Anxiety, Stress and Self Criticism', *The Journal of Positive Psychology*, 3 (2008), 182–91.

Hanson, R., & Mendius, R., *Buddha's Brain: The Practical Neuroscience of Happiness, Love, and Wisdom* (Oakland, CA: New Harbinger, 2009).

Hayes, S. C., Luoma, J., Bond, F., Masuda, A., & Lillis, J., 'Acceptance and Commitment Therapy: Model, Processes, and Outcomes', *Behaviour Research and Therapy*, 44(1), (2006), 1–25.

Henderson, L., *Improving Social Confidence and Reducing Shyness Using Compassion Focused Therapy* (Constable Robinson: London, 2010).

Hofmann, S. G., Sawyer, A. T., Witt, A. A., & Oh, D., 'The Effect of Mindfulness-Based Therapy on Anxiety and Depression: A Meta-Analytic Review', *The Journal of Consulting and Clinical Psychology*, 78, (2010), 169–83.

Jung, C. G., 'The Archetypes and the Collective Unconscious', in *Collected Works of C. G. Jung* Vol. 9, Part 1, (New Jersey: Princeton University Press, 1934).

Kabat-Zinn, J., *Wherever You Go, There You Are: Mindfulness Meditation in Everyday Life* (New York: Hyperion, 1994).

Kabat-Zinn, J., *Coming to Our Senses: Healing Ourselves and the World through Mindfulness* (New York: Piatkus, 2005).

Kritikos P. G., & Papadaki, S. P., 'The Early History of the Poppy and Opium', *Journal of the Archaeological Society of Athens*, (1967).

Kornfield, J., *A Path with Heart* (New York: Bantam Books, 1993).

Lazar, S. W., Kerr, C. E., Wasserman, R. H., Gray, J. R., Greve, D. N., Treadway, M. T., et al., 'Meditation Experience is Associated with Increased Cortical Thickness', *Neuroreport*, 16(17), (2005), 1893–7.

Leahy, R. L., *Anxiety Free* (New York: Hay House, 2010).

Linehan, M. M., *Cognitive Behavioral Treatment of Borderline Personality Disorder* (New York: Guilford, 1993).

Longe, O., Maratos, F. A., Gilbert, P., Evans, G., Volker, F., Rockliff, H. & Rippon, G., 'Having a Word with Yourself: Neural Correlates of Self-Criticism and Self-Reassurance', *Neuroimage*, 49(2), (2010), 1849–56.

Lutz, A., Brefcyznski-Lewis, J., Johnstone, T., & Davidson, R. J., 'Regulation of the Neural Circuitry of Emotion by Compassion Meditation: Effects of Meditative Expertise', *Public Library of Science*, 3, (2008), 1–5.

Mingyur Rinpoche, Y., *The Joy of Living: Unlocking the Secret and Science of Happiness* (New York: Harmony Books, 2007).

Mikulincer, M., & Shaver, P. R., *Attachment in Adulthood: Structure, Dynamics and Change* (New York: Guilford, 2007).

Neff, K. D., *Self-Compassion: Stop Beating Yourself Up and Leave Insecurity Behind* (New York: William Morrow, 2011).

Rahula, W., *What the Buddha Taught* (New York: Grove Press, 1959).

Raven, P. H., & Johnson, G. B., *Biology*, 5th Edition (Boston: McGraw-Hill Companies, 1999).

Salzberg, S., *Lovingkindness: The Revolutionary Art of Happiness* (Boston: Shambhala Publications, 1995).

Segal, Z. V., Williams, J. M. G., & Teasdale, J. D., *Mindfulness-Based Cognitive Therapy for Depression: A New Approach to Preventing Relapse* (New York: Guilford, 2002).

Siegel, D. J., *The Developing Mind* (New York: The Guilford Press, 1999).

Siegel, D. J., *The Mindful Brain* (New York: Norton, 2007).

Tirch, D., 'Mindfulness as a Context for the Cultivation for Compassion', *International Journal of Cognitive Psychotherapy*, 3, (2010), 113–23.

Tirch, D. D., & Leahy, R. L., 'Anxiety and Our Relationship to Emotional Experience: The Role of Emotional Schemas, Psychological Flexibility and Mindfulness'. Paper presented at the International Congress of Cognitive Psychotherapy, Istanbul (June, 2011).

Tirch, D. D., Leahy, R. L., & Silberstein, L., 'Relationships Among Emotional Schemas, Psychological Flexibility, Dispositional Mindfulness, and Emotion Regulation'. Paper presented at the meeting of the Association for Behavioral and Cognitive Therapies, New York (November, 2009).

Williams, M., Teasdale, J., Segal, Z., & Kabat-Zinn, J., *The Mindful Way through Depression* (New York: The Guilford Press, 2007).

Wilson, D. S., & Wilson, E. O., 'Rethinking the Theoretical Foundation of Sociobiology', *Quarterly Review of Biology*, 82(4), 327–48.

Wilson, K. G., & DuFrene, T., *Mindfulness for Two: An Acceptance and Commitment-Therapy Approach to Mindfulness in Psychotherapy* (Oakland, CA: New Harbinger, 2009).

Web Resources

My own website has many links to web resources on compassion, mindfulness and acceptance, as well as audio exercises for the practices in this book. You can reach it at:

www.mindfulcompassion.com

The Compassionate Mind Foundation is a wonderful resource for all of the great work that is going on in CFT. Their website is:

www.compassionatemind.co.uk

Dr Kristin Neff's website is another great resource for compassion focused work. It is:

www.self-compassion.org

Lastly, Dr Chris Germer has a large variety of resources available at his website:

www.mindfulselfcompassion.org

Index

The Compassionate Mind

by
Paul Gilbert

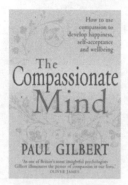

ISBN 978-1-84901-098-6
Price: £9.99

We have known for some time that developing compassion for oneself and others can help us face up to and win through hardship and find a sense of inner peace. In modern societies, however, we rarely focus on this key process that underpins successful coping and happiness and can be quick to dismiss the impact of modern living on our minds and well-being. Instead we concentrate on 'doing, achieving and having'. Now, bestselling author and leading authority on depression Professor Paul Gilbert explains that new research shows how we can all learn to develop compassion for ourselves and others and derive the benefits of this age-old wisdom.

In this groundbreaking new book he explores how our minds have developed to be highly sensitive and quick to react to perceived threats, and how this fast-acting threat-response system can be a source of anxiety, depression and aggression. He describes how studies have also shown that developing kindness and compassion for self and others can help in calming down the threat system; as a mother's care and love can soothe a baby's distress, so we can learn how to soothe ourselves.

Professor Gilbert outlines the latest findings about the value of compassion and how it works, and takes readers through basic mind-training exercises to enhance the capacity for, and use of, compassion.

Improving Social Confidence
and
Reducing Shyness

by
Lynne Henderson

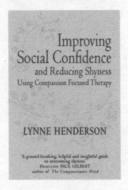

ISBN 978-1-84901-202-7
Price: £15.00

A new approach to increase confidence and
overcome problematic shyness.

Shyness can affect most of us to varying degrees, and tends to affect
children more than adults. It is a universal emotion but for some people it
develops into a more pronounced personality trait.

Shyness has evolved as an emotion over thousands of years and can
even be helpful in some circumstances – for example, when it makes
us cautious. Normal shyness, however, can become chronic thanks
to negative thoughts, avoidance and withdrawal. While shyness has
its functions, it becomes a problem when it interferes with life goals,
develops into social anxiety disorder or leads on to 'learned pessimism',
mild depression and even 'learned helplessness'.

This self-help book, based on the groundbreaking Compassion Focused
Therapy, sets out the background to shyness – its evolutionary functions,
why it becomes chronic in some people – and sets out skills and exercises
based on CFT to help the reader overcome problematic shyness.

The Compassionate Mind Approach to Beating Overeating

by
Kenneth Goss

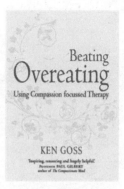

ISBN 978-1-84529-877-7
Price: £15.00

This self-help book explores the problems created by having ready access to high-fat foods designed to taste good. Because we evolved in conditions of relative scarcity we have few natural food inhibitors and so most diet books try to encourage people to inhibit their eating by highly rule-governed behaviours that have to be constantly worked at. However, this can lead to various forms of self-criticism that can undermine efforts at self-control. As a result, our relationship with eating can be complex, multifaceted and problematic.

This book uses Compassion Focused Therapy – a groundbreaking therapeutic approach – to understand and work with our urges and passions for food. We can learn to enjoy and accept food and pay attention to our biological and emotional needs. This book is for people who have tried diets and found that they don't work, and will enable the reader to have a healthier and happier relationship with food and their body.

Coming soon in the Compassionate Mind series . . .

The Compassionate Mind Approach to Managing Your Anger

by
Russell Kolts

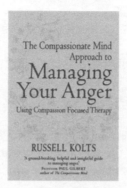

ISBN 978-1-84901-559-2
Price: £15.00

Anger is one of the most difficult emotions for human beings to cope with. When it gets hold of us we can end up behaving in extremely destructive ways towards both ourselves and other people. Under its influence we may find ourselves reacting impulsively, quietly brooding, or feeling resentful and frustrated. We often use our anger in retaliation at someone else's behaviour or to make them feel bad.

Far from 'letting you off the hook', recent research has shown that by developing compassion towards ourselves and others and understanding what drives our anger, we can develop the courage to change our behaviour. This fascinating and practical self-help guide will enable you to tackle your anger head on and take control of it, rather than letting it control you.

Dr Russell Kolts is a licensed clinical psychologist and professor at Eastern Washington University, USA. He has many years' experience in treating anger problems and has pioneered the use of Compassion Focused Therapy in working with anger, which he applies in private practice and in prison settings.

Series Editor Professor Paul Gilbert is world-renowned for his work on depression, shame and self-criticism. He is the author of *The Compassionate Mind* and integrated the techniques used in Compassion Focused Therapy.

The Compassionate Mind Approach to Building Self-Confidence

by
Mary Welford

ISBN 978-1-78033-032-7
Price: £15.00

Written by a leading expert in the field, this self-help book sets out to help the reader recognize the ways in which they are self-critical and to understand the impact this may be having on their life.

Based on groundbreaking Compassion Focused Therapy (CFT), the reader will learn proven techniques that will help them to improve their self-confidence and fulfil their goals and aspirations.

Consistent with the ethos of the Compassionate Mind Approach and the needs of the reader, this book includes findings from the latest scientific research on self-confidence and self-esteem, practical advice and a wealth of exercises.

The Compassionate Mind Approach to Recovering from Trauma

by
Deborah Lee with Sophie James

ISBN 978-1-84901-321-8
Price: £15.00

Terrible events can be very hard to deal with and those who go through trauma often feel permanently changed by it. Grief, numbness, anger, anxiety and shame are all very common emotional reactions to traumatic incidents such as an accident, or death of a loved one, or ongoing traumatic events such as domestic abuse.

How we deal with the aftermath of trauma and our own emotional response can determine how quickly we are able to 'move on' and get back to 'normality' once more. An integral part of the recovery process is not only recognizing and accepting how our lives may have been changed, but also learning to deal with feelings of shame – an extremely common reaction to trauma.

This book uses Compassion Focused Therapy to help the reader to not only develop a fuller understanding of how we react to trauma, but also to deal with any feelings of shame and start to overcome any trauma-related difficulties.

The Compassionate Mind Approach to Reducing Stress

by
Maureen Cooper

ISBN 978-1-84901-201-0
Price: £15.00

Stress is an integral part of life and something that affects us all to different degrees depending on the circumstances. It can result from trivial events such as losing your car keys, to extreme life events such as divorce, losing a child or serious illness. Each of us responds to stress in different ways, and while our body and mind responses have evolved over thousands of years and can at times be very helpful, they can also be extremely unconstructive, exacerbating already stressful situations.

Most of us have a clear understanding of the first phase of our stress response – we feel a rush of adrenaline and cortisol. However, we don't necessarily fully understand the second and third phases of our reaction to stress – actively coping with and doing things to deal with the stress, and, if the stress continues, becoming chronically stressed with high levels of arousal, making us vulnerable to feelings of anxiety, depression, irritability and fatigue.

Our understanding of the function of stress and how we go about dealing with it is intrinsically linked, and a lack of understanding can lead to bad coping mechanisms. We know our environments can cause us stress, but so does how we view stress and our ability to cope with it.

This book uses Compassion Focused Therapy to help the reader to not only develop a deeper understanding of how we all respond to stress, but also of their own individual response to stress, enabling them to spot and reverse the downward spiral into anxiety, frustration and dissatisfaction.